Rome's Ruin by Lead Poison

By the Same Author

Inventing the Ship
(Chicago, Follett Publishing Co., 1935). Exemplifies its 38 principles thru consideration of all the more important inventions in the history of the merchant ship. 294 pp.

The Sociology of Invention
(Cambridge, Mass., Massachusetts Institute of Technology, 1970). First published in 1935 as a companion volume to the above book. Examines the social principles affecting invention, both as to causation and results. 190 pp.

Social Implications of Technical Advance
Entire No. 4 of UNESCO's *Current Sociology (La sociologie contemporaine)*, vol. 1, 1953, 81 pp. With bilingual introduction by Ogburn, article of 16 pp., French summary, and annotated bib. of 55 pp. by Gilfillan and A. B. Stafford, under 30 bilingual headings, esp. of 1945-1953 works.

Invention and the Patent System
(Washington, D.C., Government Printing Office, 1964). Includes statistics of American inventive activities 1880-1960 and chapters on psychology of invention and inventors, 247 pp.

Supplement to the Sociology of Invention
(San Francisco Press, 547 Howard Street, San Francisco, CA 94105, 1971). Update on latest findings. Invention has been profoundly altered since 1935. Includes history of the inventive craft, bibliography on nature of invention, and list of periodicals. 230 pp.

ROME'S RUIN BY LEAD POISON

by

S. COLUM GILFILLAN, PhD.

Editor's note: The author has had a life-long interest in "reform spelling," so we agreed to keep some of his reforms in this book, namely, "thru," "altho," "thot" and "brot."

A short while after completing his book, the author died at age 97 in 1987, therefore this book is being published posthumously.

Library of Congress Cataloging in Publication Data

Gilfillan, S. Colum, 1889—
Rome's ruin by lead poison, by S. Colum Gilfillan.
   p.   ca.
Includes bibliographical references.
ISBN 0-930887-02-6
1. Lead—Toxicology—Rome—History
2. Rome—Nobility—Health and hygiene.
I. Title.
RA1231.L4G55 1990
615.9'25688' 09376—dc20

Library of Congress Catalog Card Number: 84-51627

Write for a free catalog to:
WENZEL PRESS
P. O. Box 14789
Long Beach, CA 90803

$Pb \cdot ♀ \cdot S \longrightarrow SPQR\text{-}S$

A puzzle, interesting and not too hard,
which tells the thesis of this book
without using a word.

Contents

Plates

Appendices

Foreword

by Clair C. Patterson, PhD, Professor of Geochemistry,
Division of Geological and Planetary Sciences
California Institute of Technology, Pasadena

Gibbon's proposed association between the downfall of the Roman Empire and the rise of Christianity was a scholarly masterpiece of the 18th century which focused widespread interest among later academicians on a central social issue. During the last two centuries classicists and sociologists have proposed many different reasons for the fall of Rome, each seeking a share of the attention initiated by Gibbon to be directed to their sociological concepts. Colum Gilfillan's proposed association between lead poisoning and the decline of Rome's genius (not its fall), formulated in the mid-20th century, is the instigator of the growth of widespread interest in lead poisoning of Romans, and this limelight situation is quite different from the sequestered context in which scholarly theories for the demise of Rome were received during the previous century.

Gilfillan grew up and was educated as a sociologist during an era when sociologists, misunderstanding the social implications of a science of evolution that was in its juvenile stage of development, commonly assumed that differences between more "advanced" cultures and those less "advanced" reflected corresponding intellectual differences between "superior" and "inferior" races. Common in their works are such statements as those by the Oxford geneticist-sociologist Darlington: "the superiority of the (extant) hunter-collector . . . (in his possession of) extraordinary perceptual faculties . . . over civilized man in what concerns his own survival is unquestionable. It is a genetic superiority for which no training can compensate. But equally he is (genetically) inferior in certain respects necessary for civilized life . . . (e.g.) he finds

i

counting difficult . . ."[1]

Darlington was among those who believed that the Roman Empire was built by a small, inbred class who possessed special aptitudes particularly suited to that purpose, but who lacked the additional and different aptitudes required to properly maintain the Empire, after its construction, in the face of new social challenges engendered by its existence. Darlington believed that Rome fell because the racial purity of the class of people who built it remained too pure through culturally determined inbreeding, and who were unable, because of cultural forbiddance, to obtain, through mixed breeding from outside sources, the genetic attributes required to meet the new and different challenges originating from and developing within an existing Empire.[2]

This same axiom of genetic racial purity, erroneously assumed to be valid in its application for sociological purposes, is used in a different interpretation to arrive at a precisely opposite viewpoint by Sir William Cecil Dampier. He believed that "swarms of alien immigrants corrupted the purity of the (ruling Roman) race, and the fall in the birthrate among the nobler and abler stocks, together with the constant drain of incessant wars . . . lowered the average quality of the . . . races which in Greece and Rome had effected such great things in the history of the world . . . (so that they) gave place to mongrel, cross-bred populations . . . fated to inward decay by their lack of cohesion, want of common ideals and disregard of statecraft . . . to (the) outward destruction . . . (and) overthrow of Rome . . ."[3]

It was into such a context of scholarly thinking and writing that Gilfillan introduced in the 1950's a truly revolutionary concept he developed from an idea of Rudolf Kobert published in 1909. Kobert's concept was that lead poisoning was probably widespread among ancient people, including Romans. Gilfillan's bombshell was a scientifically defended argument which assigned a selective lead poisoning effect to the Roman nobility, but not to the Roman poor, as the primary material cause of the inability of Rome's nobler stocks to reproduce themselves. The main effect of this new concept was not that it tended to bestow an aura of scientific respectability on such postulates as those of Sir William's, but that it stimulated many investigators to carry out new studies of lead levels in bones of both Romans and other ancient people in efforts to see whether, in fact, substantial numbers of those persons had been poisoned by lead through unsuspected means thousands of years ago. Although Gilfillan began publishing his argument in the 1950's, it did not receive widespread recognition until it was published in the *Journal of Occupational Medicine* in 1965.[4]

Gilfillan set about getting analytical evidence to support his argument by collecting bones from burials of rich and poor Romans and having them analyzed. At first he had Robert Kehoe of the University of Cincinnati Kettering Laboratory analyze some of them for lead. Kehoe, a medical advisor for and protagonist of the Ethyl Corporation, was one of my bitterest antongonists.

At that time my investigations with M. Tatsumoto and T. J. Chow of lead in the earth's oceans had disclosed the probability that lead from gasoline exhausts were polluting the entire earth through atmospheric transport. The existence of the Ethyl Corporation was threatened by my theories concerning the existence of widespread lead poisoning among Americans caused by leaded gasoline. When my colleagues and I succeeded in discovering later that the earth's oceans, atmosphere and biosphere were indeed seriously polluted with industrial lead on a global scale, this gave my laboratory a notoriety that was noticed by Gilfillan. Being passionately devoted to scholarship, Gilfillan was totally unconcerned with the niceties of feelings among opposing investigators, and immediately shifted, without a qualm, his attention to my laboratory as a more reliable source of analytical data for lead in his Roman bone samples.

The lead in bone data Gilfillan received from my Caltech (CIT) laboratory during those years were obtained at the earliest stage of development of techniques for determining concentrations of biological lead in buried human bones (which is only a minor fraction of the total lead in them). Thus, the reliability of scientific meanings ascribed to his CIT data is less than that assigned to recent lead in bone data

generated in the same laboratory by new, extremely sophisticated and highly reliable techniques which were developed
through the years after Gilfillan's samples had been analyzed.
These new techniques measure and make reliable corrections
for non-biologic lead added to the bones during burial. This
is done by determining variations in relative additions of
diagenetic lead and barium to the systematically different-
sized apatite crystals which occur in tooth enamel, compact
osseous tissue in long bone, and trabicular osseous tissue in
rib for each individual in a burial, and inferring the biologic
portion of lead from the mathematical pattern of results.
Such corrections (for diagenetically-added lead originating
from soil moisture) vary from 80% to 98% of the total lead
found in bone fragments after they have been meticulously
ultra-cleaned and selected under the binocular microscope to
remove lead contamination (which can be extremely large in
bones of people who lived in ancient cultures that did not use
lead) from dirt and present-day industrial lead introduced by
handling.

Residues amounting to only 20% to 2% of the total lead
found in carefully cleaned fragments from buried bones are
thus assigned to the biologic portion originally present in the
bones at the death of the subject. Such new techniques have
been applied to studies of bones of ancient New World
Indians and to autopsy specimens from present-day Americans to show that biologic lead levels in our ancient ancestors
used to be about a thousandth of those existing in average
Americans today.[5] Those cleaning methods used to isolate
fragments for analyses were not applied to Gilfillan's CIT
samples, nor were they analyzed (with barium) in the three
types of osseous tissue.

Gilfillan used his early CIT data to prepare a manuscript
for a book, but it was not published before he died. Word
got around about his data, however, and other investigators
immediately began to analyze lead in Roman bones so that a
number of publications on the subject now exist in the scientific literature. None of the data in those later papers possess
a quality of scientific meaning equal to even that primitive
quality in the early data obtained by CIT for Gilfillan and

presented in this book however, because later investigators have continued to use even poorer control and lack of proper consideration of lead contamination and diagenetic effects from soil and of lead contamination from sample handling and analysis. They have not attempted to use corrections of any sort.

I have not applied the new techniques to a restudy of lead in Roman bones, and it seems that other investigators attempting to carry out restudies will refuse to use the new techniques. I reviewed a manuscript of a recent major study of lead in Roman bones that will soon be published in a leading scientific journal, reporting new large-scale work on the subject, authored by a consortium of investigators from a number of universities in the U.S. and Italy. The authors use the same old inadequate analytical approaches that have been used in the past which provide lead in buried bone data whose meaning is ambiguous with respect to proportions of biologic and diagenetic lead, even though they know such methods have been replaced by new ones which can provide reliable answers. They do so because it is easier to continue with the old, simple ways—the new techniques are more difficult and require more care, time and money to carry out. Consequently, the significance and importance of their work, even though it will appear many years after the Gilfillan data were obtained, will remain small conpared to that given in this book, and will not constitute a significant advance in our scientific knowledge of the matter. Perhaps we too are living during a period of decline—one of modern science.

Although I published a statement (based on a correct evaluation of a study by other investigators who had misinterpreted their results) that Romans in Britain were probably exposed to slightly lower levels of intake of industrial lead (rather than the excessively larger levels of intake imputed by the authors) than are people in modern England exposed to today,[6] this is probably not true for Romans living in Italy where lead pollution of food and drink was higher. Colum Gilfillan believed it probable, and I believe it possible, that typical rich Romans in Italy were exposed to greater levels of lead intake than those that are typical for modern

Europeans today, with the consequence that lead poisoning in acute, life-threatening, debilitating forms were probably, or may have been, commonplace among the former. This is possible because average persons today contain such large excesses of industrial lead in their bodies (1000-fold above natural levels) that their lead intakes need only to be increased an additional 3- to 6-fold to afflict them with acute life-threatening forms of lead poisoning commonly recognized by medical clinicians.

Colum Gilfillan's creative argument concerning lead poisoning among Romans had stimulated interest in widening circles of continuing investigations into an important matter. A direct product of that stimulation is one of my arguments that the fall of Rome resulted from the loss of silver, with the resulting inflation and chaos, due to the exhaustion of lead/silver mines.[7] Gilfillan's argument will yield valuable new insights into the history of our cultural development and provide us with a new kind of knowledge about ourselves which can be used to formulate better ways for humans to live.

1. Darlington, C.D.: *The Evolution of Man and Society*, Simon and Schuster, 1969, pp. 29-30 (U.S. reprint)
2. Darlington, pp. 282-289.
3. Sir William Cecil Dampier: *A History of Science and Its Relations with Philosophy and Religion*, Cambridge University Press, 1944, pp. 75.
4. See the note on page 6.
5. Mirela Manea-Krichten, C. Patterson, G. Miller & D. Settle: Comparative increases of lead and barium with age in human tooth enamel, rib and ulna. Submitted to *Archives of Environmental Health*, 1989.
6. Patterson, C.C., Shirahata, H., Ericson, J. E., 1987. Lead in ancient human bones and its relevance to historical developments of social problems with lead, *Sci. Total Environ.*, 61:167-200.
7. Patterson, Clair C.: Silver Stocks and Losses in Ancient and Medieval Times; *Econ. Hist. Rev.*, 2nd ser., 25:205-35, 1972. And corrected modifications of these calculations are given in: Settle, D. M., and Patterson, C.C., 1980, Lead in albacore: guide to lead pollution in Americans; *Science*, 207:1167-1176.

Preface

The histories of Greece and Rome have occupied such a large part of our social thinking about the story of mankind that it is important that the major factor of Rome's ruining, and presumably of the intellectual eclipse of Greece, be discovered and set forth. The chief causal factor was above all the hitherto unsuspected bane of *lead poisoning*. But there were also certain factors of male heating, and both of these factors decimated especially the *upper, managing class.* Our imperative need for knowledge of these matters is the reason for this book.

In researching and writing it, as well as for editorial assistance, I have been especially indebted to my friend Nathaniel Weyl, a brilliant scholar and writer on our social problems. Chapters 3, 10 and 12 are mostly of his writing. Doctor Bruce E. Johnson in our medical Chapter 7, and the classical scholars Stephen N. Reinert in Chapters 10 and 11, and D. S. Godunov in Chapters 4 and 5, were engaged by me and are entitled to much thanks for their research and writing. But for all statements in this book, as finally edited, I alone am responsible.

S. Colum Gilfillan

1

The Thesis of This Book

What mattered most about the ruin of Rome was not the Empire's military defeat and breakup; those might possibly have been benefits for mankind. What concerns us here is the *decay* of Rome, the declines of genius and of every aspect of her civilization except technology, the disappearance of science after the second century, the retreat from almost all that had spelled "the glory that was Greece, and the grandeur that was Rome." There are many indications that Greece had been smitten in the same way a few centuries earlier, when her genius suddenly declined, along with her population, and that it was the importation of Greek leaded wine-making, cookery, lead face powder, very hot bathing, etc., into Rome's aristocracy around 150 B.C. that chiefly destroyed her elite, but hurt the masses too. However, the *proof* for Greece is left for some better Greek scholar.

Here is a new explanation for that decay, that intellectual ruin. It is derived not from the airy realm of the philosophy of history, but from such reliable sources as toxicology, chemistry, vital statistics and archeology, and from evidence provided by old Roman recipes and leaden pots for brewing slow poison, esteemed as delicious by the aristocracy. Our newest evidence is also archeological, from the *bones* of ancient rich and poor. Analyzed for lead, these reveal levels of the noxious metal that could have destroyed the health, mentality and fertility especially of the upper class, poisonings which they and their physicians knew little about.

We are well aware that the decay and the Fall of Rome have been favorite themes not only for professional philosophers of history, but for any curbstone amateur, and that each tends to ascribe that downfall to some evil that he op-

1

poses today. And we know especially that the *Fall* of Rome was really the net result of many causes, such as the rising strength of the barbarians, and that they were salutary as well as destructive forces. A true explanation of the ruin would have to include these all, as we explain in Chapter 14, and not just lead poisoning, the conclusive sinker that lay in the balance. All those perils of reasoning and past fiascos we know about; and therefore this our new thesis had better be good. It must be proved to the hilt. It shall be.

The Steps of Our Argument

Our argument involves the chain of facts listed below. Those already proved by familiar and conclusive evidence are followed by the letter F, and admit of brief treatment. Facts not well known but already proved by specialized authorities, are marked S; they are set forth with sufficient documentation and argued with enough cogency, we hope, to prove their import. The major ideas that have been personally added and that give our thesis its unique dysgenic import, are marked G (for Gilfillan et al) and will be developed as necessary.

1. Roman culture and every evidence of genius lost progressiveness and declined, except technology. F

2. Rome's cultural progress, aside from technology, depended on her upper class. F

3. The Roman upper class, beginning about the second century B.C., died out with extreme rapidity, each generation perhaps a third of the previous one, as a result of the well-to-do rearing very few legitimate children, and having a high mortality. S

4. All the possible causes for this extermination are examined, including political proscriptions, long hot bathing by men of leisure, change of their costume. S, G

5. And above all, lead poisoning in the upper class Romans, including their wives and mistresses, chiefly because their diet became full of lead, after the introduction of Greek cookery and abundant wine around 150 B.C. The most significant sources of lead were vintage wines, grape syrup, cooked fruits, vinegar, lead-glazed art pottery, the water

supply from lead conduits, roofs and tanks, and from lead in cosmetics, writing materials, toys and wall paint. S

6. Lead, especially in women and children, produces sterility, miscarriage, stillbirth, premature birth, severe child mortality, and permanent mental or physical impairment in children. And for all ages and both sexes, it brings emaciation, partial paralysis, gout, blindness, insanity or death. It reduces fertility in men as well. S

7. So lead poisoning was sufficient to produce the observed decimation of the upper class. And nothing else was enough. G

8. The Roman poor received some lead, but less than the rich, since they could not afford the vintage wines, grape syrup or other foods of the rich. But any sickness they suffered was a further loss to Rome. G

9. The poor had other checks to their reproduction, especially poverty, and interference with slave reproduction. F

10. Despite these unfavorable conditions the poor must have maintained their numbers without *great* decline, since the Roman population as a whole did. F

11. From items 3-7 it would follow that whatever qualities enabled Roman individuals to earn much wealth, or to grab it, keep it, marry it, or to share a rich man's board as well as his bed, were rigorously bred out of the race by lead and other forces. G

12. Industrial invention was anciently confined to the artisan class, aside from architecture, civil engineering, the art of war and agriculture. So invention continued, albeit retarded, and the use of previous inventions was hardly affected. F

13. The able son of a slave or peasant might succeed to a vacant post of leadership, but he could hardly acquire the *higher* education, family traditions nor prestige of the aristocratic scion, especially in an age of few scholarships and very expensive reading matter. F

14. In short, Roman culture lost its source of progress when and because its elite, endowed by heredity and/or upbringing with the powers to get money, was exterminated by various factors here explained, above all by lead. G

The System of Notes

It is now necessary to discuss the system of notes used in this book. Two different kinds of notes are numbered in a single series. Those notes which continue a discussion are placed at the foot of the page and referred to in the text by italic numerals, thus.[22]

Less interesting notes, usually citations, are assembled at the back of each chapter. Their indication in the text is by erect superior numerals, thus.[22]

A third class of notes involves references to our most useful or approved sources, such as Pliny's ancient encyclopedia, or to L. G. Stevenson's unequaled *History of Lead Poisoning.* We distinguish these by an asterisk* after the single name. We call them our *Starred References*, and describe each at some length in our Appendix F.

Why This Discovery Was Not Made Earlier

That the Romans must have been often lead poisoned was perceived at least as long ago as 1783, by the German Johann Beckmann, the first great historian of technology. Ancient literary evidence for lead poisoning was again pointed out in 1839 by Tanquerel des Planches* who established the modern scientific study of lead poisoning. In 1883 an Austrian professor of medical chemistry, Karl B. Hofmann,* followed by the German toxicologist Rudolf Kobert* from 1887 to 1909, well explained the ancient plague of lead by abundant citations from Greek and Roman authors on ancient culinary and dietary customs, and by illnesses historically described; and they cited archeological survivals of leaden containers for food and drink. Kobert's student Rosenblatt* analyzed ancient bones for lead and found the saturnine metal in those from the classical period, and not before nor after. More recently the physicians Lloyd G. Stevenson* and C. P. McCord[1] have written in English on the history of lead poisoning, adding further medical explanations.

Yet almost all the modern histories of medicine make no mention of lead, nor do any histories of Rome that we

have seen. We have had to rely especially on the able and ex-
haustive works of Hofmann,* Kobert* and Stevenson,* repeatedly verified by ourself and our assistance from ancient
literary sources, and from analyses we have had made from
bones of ancient people, rich and poor. Our analysts have
had the use of techniques far superior to those of Rosenblatt,* who in 1905 found no lead in some cases and could
only attest a trace of it in others. A few other works from
time to time, such as an 1824 history of wine, and Alb.
Neuburger[2] and L. S. de Camp,[3] have reported findings on
ancient lead poisoning.

And yet all those proofs of severe ancient plumbism
(lead poisoning), in the 94 years since Hofmann* and 194
since Beckmann, attracted scarcely a ripple of attention, until our first publications in 1962 and especially in 1965. The
latter attracted immense attention worldwide, as described in
the next section below. The reason is that all the students
before then had missed the *class angle*,[4] which gives to ancient
lead poisoning its great interest and social significance.

If the Greeks and Romans were lead poisoned, what of
it?, one could ask. They did not die out, and the readers had
not heard of their being sickly. But if we perceive that all the
rich Romans and their tablemates were by lead's poison left
with few children and that those were often sickly, insane, or
doomed to a short life, thus leaving most of the management
and progress of civilization to people inheriting less capacity,
wealth and education, this illuminates the famous problem of
the declines of the Greek and Roman cultures, and casts a
revealing light upon similar processes today threatening our
country and world. The present writer was able to perceive
this class angle (which all his predecessors had missed) thru
his being a sociologist of invention, a student of technic history, and an eugenist. Such a combination of social with
technological studies and interests has been a most unusual

---

4. To be sure, Hofmann spoke of the lead poison—at least in the better-
off class—and Kobert mentioned the infertility of the nobility. But
neither author, nor anyone before us, went on to find out how much
less lead the poor got, nor the vast consequences that followed from
the heavy leading of the upper class. Nor the similarly disastrous
geno-cultural effects from other harms than leading.

one, but nearly his whole career has been spent on that interface.[5]

We have found in 5 languages 44 histories of wine, or articles on the ancient wines, all but two of them published later than Beckmann's proof of lead in the wines and grape syrup which he obtained from the ancients' recipes. In only five of those histories of wine was the lead in ancient wines fairly discussed, another five barely mentioned it, and 34 said nothing about this most important fact in the whole subject of ancient wines. Yet the vintage wines of the *rich* (which both ancient and modern writers considered almost exclusively) had lead put into them in as many as 14 ways, to sterilize them so they should not go sour. Little the ancients knew that they were also sterilizing themselves.

Citations of ancient writers indicating lead poisoning are listed in Note 41 of Chapter 3. And works on Roman viniculture which overlook lead are listed in Note 19 of Chapter 4.

Publicity from the Author's First Articles

The author first managed to publish this thesis in one page of *Technology and Culture* in 1962, and much more extensively in 1965 in *Mankind Quarterly* and *Journal of Occupational Medicine*.[6] From these it was reviewed in *Medical World News, Nature, Chemistry, Hälsa, der Spiegel, die Zeit, il Tempo, Time, Time International, Harper's Mag., Saturday Review* and a host of other journals, and in five successive waves of American newspaper publicity, all unsolicited, and in books by Weyl & Possony,[7] Pendell,[8] Ehrlich,[9] Chambers[10] etc., et al. And the author spoke on it at the Third International Congress of Human Genetics in 1966.

5. For those interested, a short story of his struggles with such a difficult and novel field, covering several sciences, and a voicing of his profound regrets over having taken so long about it, is told in our Appendix G, on Data about the Author.

6. A single page in *Technology & Culture* in 1962 (Vol. 3, p.86), but picked up by Lynn White and Mortimer Chambers. Then I published more extensive articles in *Mankind Qtly.* (5:131-48) and especially in *Jol. of Occupational Medicine* (7:53-60), both in Feb. 1965.

1.   C. P. McCord: Lead and Lead Piping in Early America: *Indus. Med. & Surgery*, serially in vols. 22 and 23, 1953, 4.

2.   Alb. Neuburger: *The Technical Arts and Sciences of the Ancients*, tr. from his *Technik des Altertums*, 1930, 518 pp.

3.   L. S. de Camp: *The Ancient Engineers*, 1963, Doubleday.

4.   See the note on page 5.

5.   See the note on page 6.

6.   See the note on page 6.

7.   Nathaniel Weyl & S. T. Possony: *Geography of Intellect*, 1963, Regnery Publ., 299 pp.

8.   Elmer Pendell: *Sex vs. Civilization*, 1967, Noontime Press.

9.   Paul R. Ehrlich: *The Population Bomv*, 1968, p. 63.

10.   Mortimer Chambers: *The Fall of Rome: Can It Be Explained?* Rinehart & Winston pub., 1st ed., 1963; the 2nd ed., 1970, reprints my article from *Mankind Quarterly*.

2

Some History of Lead and Its Ancient Uses

Let us start this subject as far back as possible, at the first formation of the world. However this took place, the heavier elements naturally gravitated toward the center of our planet, leaving the lighter and lightest ones on top. Here near the top, in the biosphere, life originated, with its higher species usually at the interface between ground, water, and air. So our bodies, like all the rest of life, are composed chiefly (95.6%) of four of the lightest elements—hydrogen, nitrogen, oxygen, and carbon—and practically all the rest from the somewhat heavier elements—calcium, silicon, sulfur, phosphorous, sodium, and potassium, mostly in our bones. Of the decidedly heavy elements, such as copper and lead, almost all are poisonous to us, with the notable exception of iron, which tho heavy, is so abundant in our planet that it is frequently even in its crust, visible in all reddish or yellowish earth. No one has ever found any use for lead in the body, except that a tiny bit of it has been claimed to quicken reactions and enhance perceptions, as Detlev Stöfen has cited from Russian sources. But how obtain only that tiny bit? We daily get, and the ancients got, much more. So for us and them, every additional bit of lead has probably meant an added "insult," even if this cannot be measured nor proved. Prof. Clair C. Patterson,[1] who has best pointed out and measured in this country the growing dangers of environmental lead, says more cautiously that on general analogical grounds we ought to distrust any percentage of lead in our bodies that exceeds the percentage of the element found in the earth's crust. Lead's frequency there is .003 ppm (parts per million); and this would be still less if we included in the water and air that pervade it. In any case these considerations would warrant but a few milligrams of the saturnine metal in a man's body, not 400 times more, as today. Such reasoning is supported by the universal tendency of our bodies to suffer from and exclude metals more, the heavier their atomic weights (with the exception of iron explained above).

Yet instead of about 2 milligrams of lead in a 70-kilogram man, three parts in a hundred million, which Patterson* estimates would be normal from our diet if no lead were being mined, our present body burdens of lead are about 400 times larger than in Neolithic times. Our daily typical lead absorption is about 100 times the normal, namely, about 30 micrograms of lead per person per day.[2] (Lead breathed in, from cigarettes and leaded gasoline, is particularly noxious.)

Isotopes of Lead

Lead's heaviness is eleven times that of water, and its atomic weight 207 times that of hydrogen. Its chemical symbol is Pb, from the Latin *plumbum.* It has eleven isotopes, numbered 203 to 214, of which four are radioactive, Numbers 210, 211, 212, and 214. Pb 210 changes to Polonium 210, which is radioactive and apparently helps produce the lung cancer of cigarette smokers.[3] The various isotopes can be used for dating deposits of lead or of anything adjacent, for guessing the place where the lead was mined, and for medical experiments to determine whither the lead goes that was absorbed in different ways.

Saturn

Lead came to be associated with Saturn because there were seven "planets" known and seven metals, and because molten lead has the capacity to absorb other metals, including its own product silver, which reminded the Greeks of their myth about the Time god Cronos (Saturn to the Romans) devouring his offspring.

First Uses of Lead

Lead was perhaps the second of all metals to be discovered and used. Like most metals it was used first for jewelry. (Gold was probably the earliest discovered because of
its attractive shine and because it used to be fairly abundant
in certain streams.) Metallic lead is not found in nature, so it
was the first metal to be extracted from an ore. The process
simply required heat, and lead has a low melting point.[4]   A
stone ax has been found repaired with it.   The metal was
used in Anau I in Turkmenistan, at the dawn of horticulture.
And in earliest Troy, ca. 2200 B.C., archeologists have found
a leaden wire that served probably to fashion a woman's hair.
In central Turkey was found a leaden bead dating ca. 6000
B.C.[5]   Lead is known from 3800 B.C. in Egypt, and was used
for pipes in the V Dynasty. It was also used in Sumeria. Its
black ore, galena, supplied a cosmetic for Egyptian eyes, today called *kohl*. Its red oxide, minium, was used in the Ved-
ic period in India,[6] both as a medicine and as in modern
times for a cosmetic on the forehead.   Women in ancient
Greece and Rome wore it for red cheeks and lips, a dangerous practice.   The Old Testament and Homer mention lead.
For the Hittites around 2500 B.C. it was their chief metal. It
was the common medium of exchange in Assyria, between
the 15th and 11th centuries B.C., and was also employed for
mending pots and vases and for making water pipes[7] and cisterns. Red and white lead seem to have been used in Assyrian medicine, internally as well as externally.[7]   Neither Egyptian nor Indian medicine appears to have discovered and described lead poisoning, altho those countries used the metal.
The Greeks recognized lead poisoning later.

Lead's softness fitted it for writing tablets, and for lead
pencils to write on papyrus. (Our modern pencil "leads" are
only graphite, carbon, but the pencil may be covered with
lead paint dangerous for children who chew on it.) In Pompeii thin lead sheets coated the walls of some rooms of the

---

4.   Tin melts at 232°C, lead at 327, zinc (never separated deliberately
      by the ancients) at 419, silver at 961, copper at 1083, and iron at
      1535°.

wealthy; this was then painted over with dangerous red, white or gray lead paint to keep out dampness. The cheap and handy metal was used for statuettes,[8] like the *lares* and *penates*, and ones for children's use and for toys, but scarcely for serious works of art, nor any more for jewelry. The same soft and cheap metal was used for seals, tokens, tickets, amulets, medals of Christian devotion, sometimes for coins, often as an alloy of bronze or an alloy in late silver and gold coins, or for general household repairs, and for bullets from slings.

Hammered into thin sheets it covered roofs, made buckets, pipes (Plates 11 and 12 on page 74), tanks (Plate 2 on page 68), and it especially lined cisterns, where it would give its poison to the neutral rainwater, particularly when this was long stored, from winter rains thru the long, almost rainless Mediterranean summer. Most abundantly of all, it made pipes and tanks for almost any use where water exerted pressure, as we shall relate in Chapter 6.

As early as the Mycenaean Age building stones were bound together by iron clamps nested in melted lead. This was harmless; but pottery jars were similarly mended by lead clamps inside and out, extending from hole to hole like a strap, as seen in Plate 4 on page 69. Such jar mending goes back to Tiryns. But still this lead was probably screened from the wine by an all-over lining of resin.

Substitutes for Lead

The ancients had few good substitutes for lead. Other materials were either too expensive or too difficult to work. Pure lead, from its softness and low melting point (327°C), is the easiest of all metals to work by casting, welding and plating. Iron and steel were expensive to work and could not be cast, welded, rolled, nor drawn, their furnaces not being hot enough. Copper cannot be welded in air, and tin was eleven times as expensive as lead in Pliny's time. Gold and silver were so costly as to be out of the question, save for the rich who had some silverware on their tables. But in their kitchens they had lead utensils, where long, hot immersion made lead far more dangerous. Zinc, nickel and antimony the ancients used only in a few alloys, hardly with food, and they did not recognize their existence. Finally, wood for roofs, or to bake tiles, was relatively scarce and expensive.

Alloyed with Copper to Make Bronze

Lead was used in the ancient world as an almost unfailing alloy in bronze (copper-tin), and bronze cooking pots were used everywhere. (See Plate 9 on page 72.) Lead was used with copper, up to 30 percent,[9] both because it was much cheaper than tin and because it lowered the melting point and made a softer metal, easier to work; it is still so used in Japan.

Alloyed with Tin to Make Pewter

Lead and tin had a close association in Roman times, altho they are never found together in nature. They were often called by similar names, *plumbum nigrum vel album* in Latin, instead of *plumbum* versus *stannum* or *stagnum*. And altho in Greek their usual names were *molyb(d)os* for lead versus *kassiteros* for tin,[10] these might be interchanged. The two are mixed for soldering or plating, or to make pewter, which the Romans often employed for cups and other ornamental dishes, in a lead/tin proportion of about 30/70 or 20/80. The proportion of lead became much worse in the Middle Ages, even 95/5. And sometimes the ancients used an alloy with antimony, altho not recognizing its danger. Modern pewter may add to the tin/lead a little poisonous antimony, copper, and bismuth, to make an alloy still harder, and safe enough if we do not cook nor store acidic food in it.

The ancients used pewter not only for cups, but for plates (see Plate 3 on page 68), for a pap boat or a feeding flask for infants, and for medicine spoons. They never used pure tin for household purposes. And even today we allow one percent of lead in the tin plating of cans, and much more in their solder, which is pretty well shielded from our food. Yet critics have objected to these allowances in canned milk

10. Our Polyglot Glossary of Lead, which is Appendix E, may help.

for children, and have raised some objections to lead in our silverplate.

Silver and Lead

Silver in nature is usually found with lead, and Patterson estimates that 80 percent of Roman silver was derived from lead ores, normally galena, lead sulfide. And so around 2500—2000 B.C. men in the Near East invented the cupellation process for separating the two metals.[11] This should be considered one of the greatest inventions of all history, first because it gave men an indispensable metal for good money, neither too costly and scarce like gold or electrum (the natural gold-silver alloy early used) nor so cheap as to be available for counterfeiting coins, like the other metals. There was coinage from the 8th century B.C. onward.

So the cupellation process brot not only a metal for good money, but also abundant supplies of easily worked lead for countless uses, practical or baneful. After the ore had been pulverized by iron pestles in stone mortars, it was heated in crude furnaces of clay and stones to smelt it for its metal, almost all of it lead. This formed on its molten surface a layer of lead oxide that was blown away, until finally only a little metal was left. This remainder was practically pure silver, sometimes even purer than we make it today, containing only .01 percent of lead. But because the Greeks could not control the temperatures in the successive processes of roasting, smelting, liquation, and cupellation, a tenth of the lead and a third of the silver were lost in the slag.

Mining Silver and Lead

In the most famous of all "silver mines," that at Laurion near Athens, which was opened in the 6th century B.C., the lead was 99.7 percent of the metal; and similarly with other mines around the Aegean. The silver yield of the galena ore at Laurion was about 60 oz. to the ton, or 1/500.

The deadly mining and smelting processes destroyed countless thousands of the workers. Some breathed the lead-filled air above ground, from the pulverizing and smelting, while others worked underground with hammers, chisels, and wedges, in galleries less than a meter in height, dimly lit by little lamps that also exhausted the oxygen. Some ventilation however was provided by shafts specially dug for the purpose, and the air was fanned with cloths to create some circulation, or fires were lit, tho their smoke and carbon dioxide would also be dangerous.

Work under such atrocious conditions naturally led the slave miners and smelter workers to occasional revolt. During the Peloponnesian War, after the disastrous Athenian maritime expedition against Syracuse, some 2,000 slaves fled their Athenian masters and took refuge in the Spartan outpost at Decelea. So many of these fugitive slaves were from the gangs working the Laurion mines that the latter had to be closed in 413 B.C. to the great detriment of the Athenian treasury.

Why is it that Greek and Roman physicians have left us with few descriptions of occupational lead poisoning? The mines were worked by slaves or convicts, probably of the cheapest and most expendable types. Since Greek physicians relied for their livelihood on fees paid by their patients, why should they examine those penniless and remote miners, or describe their symptoms and ailments? Yet a few facts about their afflictions were recorded, such as smelter workers covering their heads with a balloon made from translucent bladders.

Gradually the mines gave out when the greatest depths then feasible were reached, since they had no good means to pump water up nor air down. The tailings were reworked, and finally the Laurion mines were abandoned in the first century B.C. Only in 1864, when far more advanced mining techniques could be applied, were they reopened. In 1913 Laurion produced two percent of the world's lead supply.[12]

Early in ancient times other silver-lead mines[13] were opened in many parts of the Mediterranean world, especially around the Aegean and in Cyprus, and in Spain where Pliny said 20,000 slaves worked at them, in Sardinia, Gaul, and (with little silver) in Britain. But gradually each mine was exhausted, the maximum workable depth having been reached in most cases. Meanwhile the supply of silver on hand was diminishing by about two percent each year, thru wear, ship-wrecks, hoardings, or being traded to the Orient for silk, etc., as Patterson has measured.[14] The production of silver in metric tons per year in the Mediterranean world rose from 25 tons per year in 350—250 B.C. to 60 in 250—150 B.C., to 100 in 150—50 B.C., to 200 in 50 B.C., then down to 100 in the second century A.D., to 30 in the third century A.D. and to 25 in the fourth century. Lead production presumably changed in much the same proportion. If the production of lead was 400 times that of silver, the annual lead production would have risen from 10,000 to 80,000 tons, and then sunk to 10,000 again by the fourth century A.D. Whatever the proportion of lead to silver, mined or lost, it is clear that millions of tons of the saturnine metal were produced. Karl Hofmann* estimates 2,100,000 tons in 300 years. And a good deal of it was eaten, drunk, or breathed by various kinds of people, with grave results.

Production sank still lower in the Dark Ages, along with less need for lead and silver, and its nadir was perhaps reached in the ninth century. Then silver/lead mines were opened near Goslar in central Germany, later in Silesia and Bohemia, and much later in Latin America, providing great new supplies. Ultimately, steam power for lifting water and ore, and for ventilation, vastly alleviated the sufferings of labor and multiplied the production of lead. Patterson* has measured the yearly output of lead by what was air-borne and deposited in the glaciers of Greenland. His measurements of the metal in its yearly layers there enabled charting of the northern hemisphere's yearly lead output, from an unmeasurable trifle in 800 B.C. to 100,000 tons annually in 1950 and to 3,500,000 tons in 1966. In modern times this metal has become very important, not only for batteries, solder, and paint on iron, but especially for leaded gasoline. From this we are breathing it constantly, in its burnt oxide and somewhat in its gaseous, organic form, from leaded gasoline. And lead breathed is far worse than lead eaten, since of the latter all but five or ten percent is promptly excreted; but from what is caught in the lungs, far more is retained.

1.   Clair C. Patterson, R. Elias & Y. Hirao: Impact of Present Levels
      of Aerosol Lead Concentration on both Natural Ecosystems and
      Humans: paper at International Conf. on Heavy Metals in the En-
      vironment: Toronto 1975; near Table 12.
2.   Patterson: Lead in the Environment: in *Lead Poisoning in Man
      and the Environment*, papers by Eva L. Jernigan et al, NY, Mss.
      Info. Cp., 1973, pp. 71-87; see 71.
3.   Studies by Dr. Geo. Wetherill et al. at Univ. of Calif. at Los
      Angeles in 1974. Also *Science*, Sept. 9, 1966, pp. 1259, 60.
4.   See the note on page 10.
5.   W. H. Pulsifer: *Notes for a History of Lead*, 1888, 395 pp., pp.
      150, 156.
6.   R. J. Forbes: *Studies in Ancient Technology*, 1st ed., vol. 9: cf.
      also vols. 8 and 5. E. J. Brill publ., Leiden. Also C. N. Bromhead:
      Mining and Quarrying in the 17th Century, in Ch. Singer ed.: *A
      History of Technology*, p. 1 ff.
7.   R. C. Thompson: *On the Chemistry of the Ancient Assyrians*,
      London, 1925, pp. 88 ff. Also Stevenson,* p. 416.
8.   Forbes, supra.
9.   Pulsifer, supra.
10.   Our Polyglot Glossary of Lead, which is Appendix E, may help.
11.   Forbes, supra.
12.   Chas. W. Merrill: *Rise and Future of the Lead Industry;* Stanford
      Univ. thesis, 1924, unpub., supplies a histograph of world lead
      production on p. 23.
13.   Forbes, supra.
14.   C. C. Patterson: Silver Stocks and Losses in Ancient and Medieval
      Times: *Econ. Hist. Rev.*, 25:205-35, 1972, Table 12. Also from
      footnote 2 above.

3

Greco-Roman Medical
Views of Lead

Acute Lead Poisoning

The ancient physicians, entirely Greek in background, and even the laity, knew that lead and its compounds were poisons when taken internally; but they had little or usually no idea of harm from mere contact with lead. Drawing, as we must assume, from extensive clinical experience, two Alexandrian medical writers of the second century B.C., Nicander and Cassius, described many of the symptoms of poisoning by white lead. Nicander noted froth on the gums and mucosa of the mouth, hiccups, nausea, acute and tormenting pains causing general delibility, coldness, and a stupefying drowsiness, followed by continuing deterioration toward coma and death.[1]

Such other classical authorities on medicine as Dioscorides,* Aëtius, and Scribonius Largus added such symptoms of acute lead poisoning as failing eyesight, increasing lassitude and dry throat.[2] Ingestion of litharge (lead monoxide), they wrote, caused feelings of heaviness, violent abdominal

2.   Stevenson,* 15-16. His unpublished doctoral dissertation on the *History of Lead Poisoning*, in 436 typed pages, at Johns Hopkins University in Baltimore in 1949, is unique, well done, and has been indispensable to us. It is the most comprehensive and authoritative source known to the present writer on the attitudes of classical physicians toward lead and its poison. It quotes repeatedly from Kobert,* Hofmann,* and from all the ancients indicating lead poisoning as we list in our Note 41.

pains, borborygmus (rumblings caused by intestinal gas), swollen limbs, skin discoloration, and burning sensations in the joints.

The recommended treatment for acute white lead poisoning was to induce vomiting at once, using any of a long list of emetics. After vomiting, the patient was to be given as much strong wine as he could drink, on the theory that this would counteract the coldness that lead brot to the heart. The patient was also to be prevented from falling asleep.[3] Similar remedies were advocated where the toxic agent had been litharge (Pbo, lead oxide), with the addition of such "drugs" as pomegranates, fat roast pork, and pigeon dung.

Part of the theory behind such medication was the belief which Aristotle had taught, that "cold" poisons acted by impairing that vital heat that came from the heart. Lead was a cooling agency, according to such medical authorities as Soranus[4] and Galen.[5] Therefore it must be counteracted by such heat-producing nutriments as wine and hot peppers.

Based on Hippocrates' work *On the Humors*, Greco-Roman medicine held that toxic substances migrate thru the body, causing secondary involvement if not evacuated in the normal way. This explained boils, abscesses, gangrene, and arthritis. Preventive therapy should be purgative.[6]

Chronic Lead Poisoning

Both Greeks and Romans also clearly recognized some of the forms of chronic lead poisoning. It was clear to all of them that the health of miners was severely impaired by their occupation, and clear to some that lead was a major cause of that condition. Xenophon noted that the region around Laurion, containing the greatest silver/lead mines of antiquity, was unhealthy.[7] And it was close to Athens. Lucretius observed that those who mined gold died young, and that the air from silver/lead mines was poisonous.[8] Strabo wrote that the mine owners "build their silver-smelting furnaces with high chimneys so that the smoke from the ore may be carried high into the air, for it is heavy and deadly."[9] This obviously referred, says Stevenson,* to the noxious fumes con-

taining the sulfide or oxide of lead.[10] Such writers as Lucan,
Statius, Pliny, and Silius Italicus referred customarily to miners as pallid.

Pliny wrote: "While roasting is in progress, all aper-
tures where vapors might escape must be sealed, else one
breathes the exhalations of the lead furnace."[11] The smel-
ters exposed workers to deadly fumes, mainly of lead oxide.
Dioscorides noted the dangers from this source, and Pliny
wrote that the workers "protected themselves against it by
covering their faces with bladders."[12] A century later, Julius
Pollux (A.D. 124—192) repeated that the miners in his day
covered their heads with bags, and protected their mouths
with animal-skin sheaths against inhalation of the deadly
dust.[13] One of the Hippocratic writers, in what some medical historians call a pioneer description of lead poisoning,
described the distended spleen, pallor, hard abdomen and difficult breathing of a sick miner.

The anemia caused by plumbism was described briefly
by Vitruvius, the great architect and engineer of the Augustan Age: "We can take example by the workers in lead, who
have complexions affected by pallor. For when, in casting,
the lead receives the current of air, the fumes from it occupy
the members of the body and thereupon rob the limbs of the
virtues of the blood."[14]

That some Roman writers regarded lead conduits for
water as dangerous to health will be pointed out in our sixth
chapter.   Vitruvius declared: "water is much more whole-
some from earthenware pipes than from lead pipes. For it
seems to be made injurious by lead, because white lead is
produced by it; and this is said to be harmful to the human
body."[14]

Palladius, writing in the fourth century A.D., confirmed
that lead pipes damage drinking water, adding: "Ceruse,
which is harmful to the human body, is a product of the at-
trition of lead."[15] And more than a century earlier, Galen,
physician to Marcus Aurelius, had condemned the use of water from lead pipes in preparing medicines, because it caused
dysentery,[16] hard constipation. But he was about the only
physician to mention the harm from a lead-water contact.

With this occasional recognition that water carried in lead pipes can be dangerous, it seems inconsistent that Roman physicians approved the boiling down of grape juice in lead cauldrons, to produce concentrated syrup. In fact, as we have seen, Columella, like many of his predecessors, recommended that grape juice be boiled in lead rather than in bronze containers, since the latter would taint the syrup with verdigris. This strange failure of Greco-Roman medical writers and physicians to perceive a danger that should have been apparent to them, was a major cause of the massive and prolonged assault from chronic lead poisoning, especially on the Roman wealthy and intellectual classes.

Use of Lead in General Medicine

Nutrition much concerned Medicine in Greece and Rome. Their medical writers often spoke of effects of drinking honey, wine substitutes, or additions made from honey, as well as about wine itself.[17] As we shall tell in our next chapter, those preparations were generally boiled down in leaden or lead-plated vessels, so that they inevitably took up the saturnine metal and poisoned somewhat its consumers.

Galen recommended wine sweetened with *sapa*, grape syrup, used in moderation, as a laxative.[18] Celsus, however, recognized that *defrutum*, another name for the same drink, had a constipating effect.[19] Based on this and other evidence, Kobert concluded that honey, *hydromel*, and *oxymel* were considered laxatives when raw, but constipating agents when cooked.[20] These contrary properties he pointed out were a result of cookery adding more of the constipating lead.

Galen also recommended placing lead plates on the backs of athletes to prevent nocturnal emissions, the theory being that the coldness of the metal would counteract the heat of sexual desire. Nero used such lead plates, Pliny says, to develop his powers as a singer. It is possible that such plates would rub some poison into sweaty skin.

Instruments made of lead were used to dilate the cervix, to insert into the vagina, uterus, or rectum, and to prevent adhesions after gynecological operations. Soranus recommended the use of leaden sounds to fumigate the uterus.[21] The effects must have been severely abortifacient. Lead is taken up very slowly in neutral water, but dissolves readily in warm acid and to a lesser extent in alkaline solutions. If the recommended fumigant should contain vinegar and be inserted with a leaden tube, as Soranus recommended, significant amounts of lead acetate would be deposited directly in the womb. This would cause abortion in young women otherwise quite capable of bearing healthy children.

The extended coverage Soranus gives to a prolapsed uterus seems highly significant in this context. This pathological condition is rare in modern times, but it was common in the Roman times. The prolapse could well have been caused by the introduction of lead in an acidic solution into the womb, causing an atomic condition there.

Catheters and bougies, which could penetrate deeply into the passages of the body either for draining or dilation, were often of lead. Leaden instruments were inserted into the vagina and rectum and were used to dilate the cervix, transmitting some of their saturnine poison.[22]

Contraception and Abortion

Lead and lead preparations played a prominent part in Greco-Roman abortifacient and gynecological practice. One of the oldest references comes from Aristotle's *History of Animals:*

> *"But if, on the contrary, we want to avoid conception, then we must bring about a contrary disposition. Wherefore, since if the parts be smooth, conception is prevented, some anoint that part of the womb on which the seed falls with oil of cedar, or with ointment of lead, or with frankincense, commingled with olive oil."*[23]

Writing four centuries later, Soranus of Ephesus, the greatest gynecologist of antiquity, recommended white lead as one possible ingredient of a contraceptive mixture to be

applied to the mouth of the womb.[24] He also suggested that
"to prevent conception, the woman before conception
should smear her cervix with rancid oil, or with honey, or
with a decoction of cedar oil, or she should push into the *os*
a thin strip of lint, or introduce into the vagina an astringent
pessary."

The contraceptive procedures recommended by Soranus
would less often fail if the astringent pessary contained lead,
or if the honey or cedar oil had been prepared with *defrutum*
(a leaded grape syrup) or in a lead-lined vessel. In the latter
case, the long-range consequence of resorting to these practices would tend toward the sterilization and possible chronic
lead poisoning of the woman.

Pliny* said that grape syrup (which had been boiled
down in lead, filling it with poison) drunk with onion "becomes a means of abortion and can be used medically to ex-
tract from the womb dead fetuses and premature births."[25]
But Kobert observed that the lead first kills the fetus and
thereby brings on its abortion.[26] He observed that onions
could not conceivably be a cause, since it is well known that
Jews eat large quantities of onions, yet produce numerous
and healthy children. The culprit therefore must be the lead
in which the grape juice was boiled down to syrup. The lead
did not merely facilitate the removal of the dead embryo, but
in fact killed it first.

An oral contraceptive called *adynamon* was a favorite
drink of prostitutes. To grape syrup, of course leaded, sea
water was added and it was again boiled, naturally in lead.
So it interfered both with conception and with normal development of a fetus. *Adynamon* was favored also for its lack
of alcohol, sobriety being a financial necessity for practitioners of the oldest profession.[27]

There is also evidence that crude sorts of condoms were
occasionally used by the Romans, and that these might contain lead preparations. Contraception's acceptance will be
discussed in Chapter 10.

Sterilizing Wounds

While all Greco-Roman medical writers opposed eating

or drinking lead or its perceived compounds, they recognized their cicatrizing properties on external sores and wounds. Lead has cooling properties, much airy substance, little earth, and is moist, Galen wrote. Hence it should be mixed with cold liquids to produce an astringent concoction that could be applied to relieve fissures, hemorrhoids, and ulcers, particularly ulcers of the joints, buttocks, and genitals.[28]

Lead sulfide and litharge were used to cicatrize wounds. These preparations were indeed highly efficient germicidal agents; and they also caused cell death around the margins of wounds, thus favoring the formation of scar tissue. Mortality from blood poisoning was extremely high until the last century. Hence any agency that effectively closed open wounds or sores was medically beneficial, despite the long-range risk of lead poisoning which its use might entail.

Soranus recommended that when no longer inflamed, the cavities of sores be filled with white lead. Dioscorides approved the use of lead salts to stop bleeding. Celsus and Pliny thot ointments of lead compounds should be applied for bites, burns, and wounds.[29]

Soranus[30] advised that infants bruised in delivery be anointed with white lead and litharge, most dangerous advice since infants are so susceptible to plumbism. Galen recommended litharge to cure interigo, an inflammation of the skin. Lead salts were also recommended for collyria, eye lotions.[31]

The Diagnosis of Lead Poisoning

Diagnosis was difficult for the Greeks and Romans, since they lacked quantitative methods of pathology, had no laboratories, and knew no chemistry. Their underlying medical science rested on false assumptions, such as Aristotle's concept of the four humors, the hot and cold, wet and dry. Diagnosis rested largely on the visual and tactile impressions of the physicians. Since ordinary lead poisoning often reaches an acute stage after contact with the infecting source has ceased, it is no wonder that the ancient physicians often failed to perceive the connection between lead and its toxic effects.

As to occupational lead poisoning, we have an enigmatic account in one of the Hippocratic writings, of a man from the mines, who suffered from abdominal swelling, enlarged spleen, tense abdomen, pallor, and respiratory difficulties. Tanquerel des Planches* considered this an early description of lead poisoning; yet Stevenson* noted that pain, constipation, and paralysis were not listed among the symptoms.[32] But part of the problem is that the symptoms of plumbism are highly varied. Yet lead's typical paralysis of the extensor muscles of the lower arm and leg was noted by Soranus and Caelius Aurelianus.

The lack of clearer and more frequent descriptions of occupational lead poisoning may be attributed to several causes. Then, as now, competent doctors much preferred to practice in the cities rather than in mining communities. Public health care was virtually nonexistent; physicians relied on patients' fees for their livelihood. From this standpoint, the miners, usually convicts or slaves, almost always near the bottom of the social pyramid, were unpromising clients. Galen boasted that he gave the same care to slaves as to senators; but no Roman physician was under compulsion to treat patients who were unable or unwilling to pay.

One of Martial's epigrams tells an interesting story, explained at the time, of optic neuritis caused by lead:

> *"Phryx, a notorious tippler, was blind of one eye, and blear-eyed in the other. Heras, his doctor, said to him: 'Beware of drinking: if you drink wine you will not see at all.' Phryx laughed, and said to his eye 'adieu.' Immediately, he orders eleven measures 'nearly three times the usual quantity' to be mixed for him, and frequently. Do you ask the result? Phryx drank a vintage, his eye venom."*[33]

Rutherford wrote convincingly in a medical journal that such blindness could not have been caused by alcohol and must have been due to lead.[34]

Hippocratic writers referred to "colic, pains about the

navel, and ache in the loins," progressing to inflammation of the abdominal wall and to colic without fever, causing heaviness of the knees and gut pains.[35] An ancient statement that these colic pains could be eased by pressure around the navel and by opium, is further confirmation of lead poisoning.

Pliny noted that epidemic colic first appeared in Italy during the reign of Tiberius, and that the Emperor himself was the first person attacked by it, "a circumstance which produced considerable mystification thruout the city, when it read the edict issued by that prince excusing his inattention to public business on the ground of his being laid up with a disease, the name of which was then unknown."[36]

It is tempting to speculate that all the emperors who seemed insane, including Nero, Caligula (a drunkard), perhaps Tiberius, in the Julio-Claudian line, and Domitian, became so thru lead encephalopathy. Caligula was certainly insane, Nero probably so, Tiberius, tho generally respected by historians, was accused by the gossipy Suetonius of extraordinary drunkenness and stupid actions thereby. His distinguished medical biographer, Gregorio Marañón, said that he was temperate except for "some excess in wine drinking, had skin diseases and fetid ulcers, and was probably impotent,"[37] Some later emperors, Commodus perhaps and Elagabalus certainly, were insane.

The ancient physicians seem to have had no idea of *Encephalopathia saturnina*, insanity from lead. Yet the common folk seem to have had some notion of it, because *Tu plumbarie*, "you crazy lead-worker," was a term of contempt, doubtless from a perception that the very numerous workers in hot lead were inclined to be crazy. Similarly, when Gilfillan was a boy there was a proverbial expression, "Crazy as a painter." It is not heard now, because that trade has become better protected and its lead mostly removed.

Of the clinical descriptions that fit the pathology of lead poisoning, the most intriguing is the epidemic described by Paulus of Aegina in the third century A.D. He wrote of a sickness that "having taken its rise in Italy, but raging also in many other regions of the Empire, like a pestilential contagion, in many cases terminates with epilepsy, but in others in paralysis of the extremities," adding that most of those with epileptoid symptoms died and most of those with paralytic ones recovered.[38] This appears, the generally skeptical Stevenson writes, "a clear description of lead poisoning."[39] Such an epidemic, raging thruout the Empire, could have been caused by an unusually bad harvest. When the wine went sour, the temptation was to sweeten and preserve it from turning to vinegar, by adding unusually large quantities of grape syrup (boiled down in lead containers).

To summarize: Greek and Roman physicians recognized that lead and its products were poisonous when taken internally. They did not recognize the medical dangers of unintended consumption of lead thru the numerous products cooked or stored in leaded containers. They also used lead and lead products extensively for surgical instruments, such as sounds and catheters, which were inserted into the vagina and womb, causing miscarriage and sterility.[40]

Lead preparations were applied to boils, ulcers, adhesions and open wounds, risking massive toxic effect. From the time of Aristotle to the last centuries of the Empire, lead was recommended in gynecology and for abortion. Thus, the medicine of the time encouraged the application of lead and lead products in forms which would contribute significantly to sterility.

These sterilizations were class selective, decimating especially the wealthy. They were the minority with access to learned medicine and to trained physicians. As for the urban proletarians and the rural poor, the great majority never saw a physician, but relied on home remedies, magical concoctions, or potions purchased from vendors called *pharmacopolae*, as they thot appropriate or could be persuaded to buy. These might be leaded or not. In large slave communities, which might number a hundred or more for a great establishment, one slave was appointed to be doctor and druggist for the rest.

We list in our Note 41 eight other citations of ancient writers on lead poisoning, from Dr. L. G. Stevenson's* very valuable but apparently unpublished dissertation, *A History of Lead Poisoning.*

1. Nicander: *Alexipharmaca*, 23-24.
2. See the note on page 17.
3. Stevenson,* pp. 18-19.
4. Soranus, *Gynaecology*, II, 41.
5. *Claudii Galeni Opera Omnia*. (Kuhn ed., Leipzig, 1821-33), XII, 31.
6. Stevenson,* 8-10.
7. Xenophon, *Memorabilia*. (Loeb edition), VI, 6, 12.
8. Lucretius, *De Rerum Natura*, VI, 811.
9. Strabo, *Geography*, III, 2, 8.
10. Stevenson,* 33-34.
11. Pliny,* XXIV, 167.
12. Pliny,* XXXIII, vii, 40.
13. Stevenson,* 36.
14. Vitruvius, *De Architectura*, VIII, 6, 11.
15. Palladius,* IX, 11. Quoted by Stevenson,* 52.
16. Galen, supra, note 5, XIII, 45.
17. T. C. Allbutt, *Greek Medicine in Rome*. (Lon., 1921), 329-330.
18. Galen,* 633.
19. A. Cornelius Celsus: *De Medicina*, in the Augustan Age, II, 29.
20. Kobert,* 105, 111. He also supplies information on lead in ancient Medicine, in his *Vorwort zu Aulus Cornelius Celsus über die Arzneiwissenschaft* in 8 Büchern übersetzt von Ed.Scheller, 1906.
21. Wm. J. S. McKay, *History of Ancient Gynecology*, 1901, pp. 99, 39, 163.
22. Soranus, *Gynaecology*, II:14.
23. Aristotle, *History of Animals*, Thompson tr. 583a, 20.
24. Soranus, *Gynaecology*, I, 61.
25. Pliny,* XXIII, 30.
26. Kobert,* p. 112.
27. Dioscorides,* 5:13 or Pliny,* XIV:16.
28. Stevenson,* 22-23.
29. Stevenson,* 25.
30. Soranus, *Gynaecology*, I:61.
31. Wm. Smith & Wayte & Marindin; *Dictionary of Greek and Roman Antiquities*, gives references on collyria.
32. Stevenson, * 37.
33. Martial, *Epistles*, VI, 78.
34. W. J. Rutherford, "Lead Poisoning in the First Century," *British Jol. of Ophthalmology*, (1934), 18:36-38.
35. Stevenson,* 87-88.
36. Pliny,* XXVI, 6.
37. Gregorio Marañón: *Tiberius: A Study in Resentment*, (London,

Hollis & Carter, 1956), 172-173.

38.   *The Seven Books of Paulus of Aegina*, Adams tr., Lon., (1844-47),
      vol. I, 396-7, 534. Quoted by Stevenson,* 90-91.

39.   Stevenson,* 91.

40.   McKay, supra.

41.   Stevenson* provides the following citations of ancient writers in-
      dicating lead poisoning:

      Nicander: *Alexipharmaca*, lines 74-114 & 594-610, from the tr.
      by M. Brenning in *Allg. Med. Central-Zeitung*, 1904, Nos. 17
      ff. pp. 368-9, 389; and reprint, pp. 23, 24, 41.

      Dioscorides,* ed. by Kuhn, II, pp. 32, 26, 337, altho this *Liber de
      Venenis* is regarded as a spurious work; (cf. Wellman in Pauly-
      Wissowa, *Real-Encyclopedie der classischen Altertumswissen-
      schaft*, V:1140; and Ernst H. F. Meyer: *Geschichte der Botanik*,
      1854-7, II:107 ff).

      Celsus: *De Medicina*, V,27, 12th ed.; Spencer II:123.

      Scribonius Largus: *Compositiones*, 183-4, ed. by G. Helmfeich,
      pp. 74-5.

      Galen,* ed. by Kuhn, VII:139, and XIV:142, 144-6.

      Aëtius of Amida: *Aëtii Medici Graeci Contractae ex Veteribus
      Medicinae Tetrabiblos*, IV, I, 78. Latin tr. by Cornarius, 1542,
      p. 712.

      Paulus of Aegina: *The Seven Books of Paulus Aegineta*, tr. by
      Francis Adams, 1844-7, II, pp. 234-8. This list extends from
      the 2nd century B.C. to the 7th A.D.

4

The Drinks and Foods
of the Rich and Poor

Wine and grape syrup were probably the most important sources of lead poisoning for the ancient Romans. The
cultivation of grapes and their precious pressed products dates
from early millennia, and came to Rome thru Greece. Pliny
wrote, "Supremacy in respect to the vine is to such a degree
the special distinction of Italy, that even with this one possession she can be thot to have conquered all the good things
of the world."[1]

But in the early centuries of the Republic, wine was regarded as something of a luxury. Lucius Lucullus recalled
that when he was a boy (around 80 B.C.) Greek wine was
never given more than one serving in his father's house. But
when he was a man he distributed 100,000 jars of Greek wine
as largesse.[2] In 46 B.C. Julius Caesar broke all precedent by
serving four different kinds of wine at a banquet.[2]

Women Prohibited from Drinking Wine

From the health and genetic standpoints, the drinking
of lead-tainted wine is much more dangerous for women than
for men, because of the greater effect it can have thru wom-
en by causing sterility, abortion, stillbirth, teratogenesis, and
neontal death.[3] In the stern earlier centuries of the Roman

---

3. And as to mere alcohol in wine, it has been known since ancient
   times that its excess, alcoholism, in pregnant women after the third
   month, is damaging to the pregnancy and fetus, producing mental
   and physical defects in the offspring. Statement of Dr. Ernest P.
   Noble, Dir. of Natl. Institute on Alcoholic Abuse and Alcoholism.

Republic, women were prohibited from drinking wine, and the rule could be savagely enforced. Pliny records that the wife of Egnatius Mecenius was clubbed to death by her husband for drinking wine, and that Romulus acquitted him. Fabius Pictor wrote in his *Annals* around 300 B.C. that a matron was starved to death by her relatives for having broken open the casket containing the keys to the wine cellar.[4] Cato observed that "the husband has an absolute authority over his wife, it is for him to punish her if she has been guilty of any shameful act, such as drinking wine or committing adultery."[5] The reason for the prohibition, according to the first century A.D. historian Valerius Maximus, was the belief that drinking women might become sexually aroused and be unfaithful. Pliny said that Roman men often kissed female relatives to find out whether they had been drinking. "The Bona Dea," Lecky tells us, "it is said, was originally a women named Fatua, who was famous for her modesty and fidelity to her husband, but who, unfortunately, having once found a jar of wine in the house, got drunk, and was in consequence scourged to death by her husband. He afterwards repented of his act and paid divine honors to her memory, and as a memorial of her death, a vessel of wine was always placed upon the altar during the rites."[6]

But those drastic punishments, which were doubtless exceptional if not fictional, dated from the misty earlier centuries of Rome. The culture of grapes, for wine chiefly, became important in central Italy by the middle of the second century B.C. Since women had higher status in the Roman than the Greek world, and were allowed to take part in banquets with their husbands, it was natural that once wine drinking became popular in the upper classes, women would also drink. Just when the old ban broke down is not clear,[7] but this likely occurred somewhere around 150 B.C. when

5.   The passage from Cato was preserved and quoted by the second century A.D. grammarian, Aulus Gellius, *Noctes*, x. 23.

7.   AElian said much about the old rules, including a permission to drink wine to noble wives over 35 (past the main childbearing age). But we found in his work no clear indications of date. *Variae Historiae*, written in Greek about 70 A.D., e.g., II:38.

Rome conquered Greece, altho Polybius still spoke of the prohibition being in force around that time.[8] And Cato (d. 149 B.C.) also noted that a husband could forbid wine to his wife. Somewhat later we find reports of female drunkenness. Sextus Propertius (49-15 B.C.) described how, when his mistress Cynthia found another lover, he invited Phyllis to a drinking party because "sober she pleases me little, when she drinks all is charm." Again he said of Teia: "fair is she, but when the wine is on her, one lover will be all too few."[9]

Martial (A.D. 60-102?) included in his gallery of heavy wine drinkers the woman Myrtale, "Flushed and with swollen veins," who was "wont to reek with too much wine." He blamed female drunkenness on too much money and on alien customs.[10]

Several ancient writers also indicate that wine in the upper class became much more common by the first two centuries B.C.

As for the common people, Ovid (43 B.C.-17 A.D.) writes of young couples picnicking and drinking wine in the countryside near the Tiber, during the New Year festival of Anna Perenna.[11] And he mentions a drunk old woman who lugged an old man in like condition.

Excessive Wine Went to the Wealthy

In the last century of the Republic and increasingly in the Empire, drunkenness seems to have become common among the upper class. Pliny* excoriated the topers who "got themselves boiled in hot baths" and were carried out of the bathing hall unconscious, with pallid cheeks. Customs arose among the rich of competitive drinking and of vomiting (a symptom of lead poisoning); but we shall write of those in our 12th chapter on the evidences of degeneration. The emperor Tiberius was a heavy drinker, as was his son Drusus Caesar. Mark Antony was famous for his drinking exploits, and was drunk the evening before he lost the decisive battle of Actium.[12]

---

8.   Polybius, *Histories*, VI:2, said they could drink *passum vinum*.

Ending his chapter 14 on wine (14:28) Pliny tells not only of prodigious drinkers, but of the ordinary drunkard's "pale face and hanging cheeks, sore eyes, shaky hands that spill . . . and condign punishments of haunted sleep and restless nights." All these are symptoms of lead poisoning. The French physician A. L. A. Fée, before 1855, remarked that the Roman wines must have been somehow different from ours, which produce red, not gray cheeks. (Gray cheeks are a symptom of the gray metal.)

From such stories we draw at least three conclusions: that some of the wine must have been vomited up, as indeed was often told, followed by drinking more, that the worst cases were exaggerated or atypical and that still the wealthiest Romans must have consumed too much wine, and got much lead from their vintage wines, grape syrup and many other foods (and other sources).

The More Temperate Poor

The poor were of necessity more temperate, and as we shall show, their wine apparently contained much less lead. But wine "formed part of the staple diet, and even slaves were allowed their ration."[13] The very poor drank a third-rate wine obtained by repressing the lees of the grapes. An early authority observed that "the drink of the Roman was water, but he mixed it with wine whenever he had the chance."[13] There were a few similar alcoholic drinks for the upper class, but beer was considered to be for barbarians or the poor. Even in the early centuries of Rome, the masses celebrated the April and August festivals of wine, called *vinaliae*. Rough wine was at times very cheap. In 250 B.C., for example, a bountiful year, ordinary wine sold for an *as* the *congius* (3.28 liters).[13]

The common people once hoped for free wine as well as free grain, but Augustus rejected this proposed extension of the *sportula* (dole). "But," said Suetonius, "to show that he was a prince who desired the public welfare rather than popularity, when the people complained of the scarcity and high price of wine, he rebuked them, saying: 'My son-in-law,

Agrippa, has taken good care by building several large aqueducts, that men shall not go thirsty.' "[14]

The extent to which Roman laborers and peasants were able to drink wine can be inferred from the relationship between their wages and its cost. In 150 B.C. ordinary wine cost about three sesterces the gallon (3.8 liters). That was the daily wage of an ordinary free laborer. A slave's labor would be valued at two sesterces. And in 89 B.C. a day's wage for unskilled labor bought 3.8 liters of common wine. Therefore considerable wine could be consumed by the poor; but it was expensive enough to make widespread and chronic alcoholism among them rare.

Diets of the Rich and Poor

The main food of the poor, as of the soldiers, was *porridge*, made by boiling various cracked grains, especially emmer and spelt (varieties of wheat), or barley, millet, or beans. And sometimes they used acorns. The boiling may have been done in a leaden, pewter, or lead-lined bronze pot, or they might have used the cheap pottery, unglazed like our terra cotta, a poor conductor of heat, but everywhere easily made from local clay. We have been unable to determine the relative frequency among the poor of such ceramic instead of plumbiferous metal pots. Archeology rarely helps because most metal pots have been salvaged, but hardly common or broken pottery. Herculaneum would be the place to search, because it was overwhelmed by a flood of mud, neither melting metals as at Pompeii nor allowing salvage. In any case where porridge was cooked in large quantities, as in a mansion housing many slaves, a larger and probably metal pot would have been used. The surface per liter would be less in a larger pot, hence giving a health advantage to the slaves.

The diet of the poor included also some bread, milk, cheese, beans, chick-peas, beets, turnips, onions, garlic, other greens, considerable dried fish but little meat, an occasional grasshopper, some fruits, beer, a little olive oil, and considerable vinegar (perhaps derived from spoiled vintage wine which might well have spoiled because it was not leaded), often taken with water *(posca)* and sometimes mixed with eggs.

The diet of the rich was more like our own, except that it included abundant wine, and in lieu of sugar much grape syrup and honey. And we think the rich would be more inclined to store and cook their foods in metal pots, pails, tanks and other containers often leaden, while the poor, especially peasants, probably used lead-free pottery or wood. Metal containers had to be either lead, pewter, or bronze, the latter always containing lead too, and preferably polished and oiled to reduce copper poisoning, or plated inside with lead or a lead-tin alloy. We have found but one record of a vessel made of pure tin.

Notably deficient in the diets of both rich and poor, at least in the cities, was milk, except in the form of cheese. And milk is an antidote for lead. (The calcium in milk is an element related to lead, that displaces it.)   The Solomon's book[15] on Roman cookery says the aristocracy did not like milk: in 96 luxury recipes which these historians modernize from Apicius,* only five contained milk, three cheese, and none butter. The reason would presumably be the difficulty of keeping milk from souring, in a warm climate with no refrigeration, bad packaging, and very slow land transport from farm to city.   Centuries later, after Rome's ruin, we find creative ability first reappearing in the sparse populations of Ireland and Iceland, whose cool and rainy climates precluded cultivation of grapes, and required a diet largely of milk and milk products.

How the Wines Were Made for the Wealthy

The Roman procedures for making wine were similar to those used by the Greeks, and both lands produced various surviving books on viniculture and enology, wine-making. Their procedures involved in the preparation of wine required so many take-ups of lead that these probably formed the greatest source of lead poisoning for the Roman upper class.

To produce wine, the Romans extracted the juice (the must) in different ways. For the best wine the grapes were piled up until their own weight squeezed out the very best juice, after which they were trodden to obtain more. Wines extracted by these methods and further treated we shall call vintage wines; they were commonly aged for a year or more and were higher priced. Next the lees, the residue from the first pressing, were doused with water and heavily pressed under a great lever beam or sometimes a screw. The small press shown in Plate 18 on page 78, operated by wedges driven in, is a more primitive contrivance, fancifully painted.[16]

For the poorest grade of wine there was a second watering and pressing. Then the lees might even be cooked, in Greek practice, which would doubtless introduce some lead for the poor. All wines would get a little lead from the collecting basin, the *lacus*, reached thru a lead pipe of course, and also often from the strainer, the *colum*. This would often be made of lead unless of wickerwork, rushes, or of cloth for a finer straining; there were no wire-woven sieves. But these leaden receptacles involved only brief lead exposure and no heat. In the press the grapes would be confined in linen bags or in baskets of woven esparto grass, which were separated by wooden slats or sometimes, we think, by perforated lead plates. While being pressed the whole mass was kept in place by ropes or straps.

A little further leading of the must would be accomplished by use of lead pails, pipes and pumps, by which the juice was usually transferred to an immense pottery jar (Latin *dolium*, Greek *pithos*[17]), the vat in which the must would

16. On the Greek writers and on Roman diet and countless other matters of ancient procedure a great source is the late Robert J. Forbes: *Studies in Ancient Technology*, 9 vol., E. J. Brill pub., London; 1st ed. 1955 (cf. vol. 3, pp. 108, 116, or cf. the 2nd ed. 1971). Here he notices Kobert,* and apparently had heard some echo of lead poison ruining Rome, which he dismissed with an exclamation point!

   A recent work is by J. & J. Solomon, note 15. Among the Greek writers on viniculture were Theophrastos, Philliston of Locri, and Athenaeus* of Naucratis. The chief Roman writers were Pliny,* Cato,* Columella* and Varro. And of course the modern historians Kobert,* Hofmann,* Stevenson* and also Soyer.*

17. It was under such a *pithos*, broken and abandoned, that Diogenes found shelter. He never saw a tub in his life; coopery was a later, northern invention. But later, barrels were used by the Romans, for storage and for land transportation in lieu of wineskins.

ferment to wine. (See Plate 4 on page 69.) But often, especially in wet years, the must was first boiled to remove excess water; and naturally such boiling would involve further leading.

Amphoras

After fermentation and often sophistication the wine was aged, occasionally for ten years, in ceramic amphoras, or, after the introduction of the northern invention, in wooden barrels. These latter might have leaden hoops, another very minor source of saturnization. A little olive oil was floated at the top of the amphora, or barrel, to shut out air. An amphora was stoppered by a ceramic plug, or later one of cork. The clay stoppers were sealed with grape syrup, resin, clay, or gypsum. Philippe Diolé tells in his *4,000 Years Under the Sea* that many amphoras have been recovered from wrecks near the Riviera, with their stoppers, but not with their wine surviving. Yet we have ourselves found lead in five of our amphoras which we had examined. (See Appendix B on page 201.)

These amphoras were two-handled ceramic vessels of varied shape, each holding 26.3 liters. (See Plates 5-7 on pages 70-71.) They might serve likewise for grape syrup, olive oil or other liquid food. For land transportation they were replaced by wineskins, or metal flagons, or else later by the coopered barrel.

If the must was of the best quality, there was no further treatment, save usually to store the amphoras in a warm, smoky room *(fumarium)* in which the wine would age for a year or more.

Correcting Wine

When the wine was not of the best quality the Roman vintners knew many tricks to improve it—or at least to hide its defects—and to vary its type. Resin or wood tar pitch lined the interior of the amphoras, giving a flavor still favored by the modern Greeks in their retzina wine. This pitch doubtless also afforded some protection against any lead clamps, inside and out, such as were often used to repair cracked amphoras and vats (Plate 4 on page 69). A great variety of herbs, flowers or minerals (salt, lime, marble, gypsum) were sometimes inserted for bouquet, flavor, or medicinal purposes, as Pliny* recounts, including the always leaded grape syrup. Again and again he (XIV:27) and Cato,* and Columella* especially (XII:26), say that "leaden and not bronze jars should be used" for boiling new wine, or the grape syrup they would so often put into the vintage wines, fancy drinks, or medicines for the upper class. And Columella would boil down seawater to one-third, as if he wanted lead chloride too, and kept it for three years (in a lead-lined cistern probably); then there would be no fear of the wine spoiling, he says in 12:21. He might also boil the wine (12:25), first adding a tenth of water and then boiling it down. Hofmann* discussed with a chemist's eye for plumbism the ways in which lead was introduced into the "good," durable wines and fruit foods, so many ways to convey lead, none of which the ancients recognized, save for very rare exceptions.

How the Lead Was Added

The Romans put lead poison into their wines and most of their "better" fruit drinks and fruit preserves in as many as fourteen ways, so that the wines would last, not go sour by further fermentation—or to make them sweeter. Another motive was to avoid *copper* poisoning, something that they knew about; it was bad for everyone but an enemy. One can even *see* it in the green verdigris, and taste it, and it produces prompt and recognized sickness. But lead poisoning, as we have said, is a snake of another color, much less visible, tasteless or mildly sweet, and years slow in acting, unless one swallowed a solid dose. And when at last its effects become evident, they are highly varied and resemble other diseases. So how could the ancients correlate those varied and delayed effects with everyday actions, practices that had been used for years, and were generally like their peers' actions?

To avoid or reduce copper poisoning without resorting

to the primitive, fouled, and heat-blocking terra cotta, the ancient upper class knew of several other methods beside the simple replacement of the (lead-)bronze pot by a leaden one. They could plate the bronze pot internally with lead, or with a lead-tin alloy. Or they could use a pewter pot (lead-tin) or pure tin; but we have never found but one mention of this last. Or they could polish the lead-bronze pot with chalk, and oil it, as some authors mention. All these methods (except the hypothetical use of pure tin) would still leave some of the lead. And a moderate amount of lead was just what they were unwittingly seeking, for various purposes, namely, for the sterilization of the fruit juice against fermentation, or for sweetness, or to combat diarrhea by its opposite, constipation.

A leaden or a lead-tin plating could be obtained by pouring this alloy molten into the pot, or more easily by heating the pot and rubbing onto it a block of the softer metal or alloy. Such means have been practiced up to modern times in Turkey, India, Pakistan, and Burma, where such plating might be renewed monthly in the marketplace. In France in 1765 the *Encyclopédie* described a 1:2 lead-tin plating by pouring *(etamage)*; no objections to the lead were stated.

Such a plating normally disappears during centuries underground, by galvanic action. But Hofmann* tells of such having been found, presumably in a dry place.

That solid lead was used often or usually, rather than lead-plated (or possibly tinned) lead-bronze, is indicated by the so frequent reference to leaden vessels ("not bronze") and by a warning against letting a pebble or a coin get in the pot, lest it cause the melting of a hole thru it. And likewise for constant stirring with a brush of twigs or fennel, when grape syrup was being boiled down, lest a baking of the syrup in some spot cause a hole to melt there.[18] No holes could be created like this unless the pot were of solid lead. The constant stirring would surely scrape off some oil and promote leading. See Plate 18 on page 78 which shows on the left the juice being boiled and stirred.

Three dissertations and a book, all on ancient vinicul-

ture and all overlooking the lead that stares a chemist in the
face, are listed in our Note 19.

Possible Substitutes for Lead

Today of course we have many alternative materials for
lead-free pots: iron, aluminum, glass, enameled ware, and
fully fired glazed and thin chinaware. But the ancients
lacked all such, save that they used glass without cooking in
it. We have, to be sure, seen three modern references[20] to an
ancient iron skillet, and pot, but doubt the authenticity of
some others. For the ancient writers hardly seem to mention
them, and certainly they never *cast* iron, since their furnaces
were not hot enough. Nor could they truly *weld* iron, but
only wrap one piece around another, because of the same
lack of heat. They could hammer a bar of red-hot iron into a
sword, knife, rod, or such shapes, and then grind it. But to
hammer out a concave skillet, much less a pot, and give it
sufficient uniformity of thickness so that it would not burn
the food in some thin spots, nor be ruined by a hole or rust-
ing, would seem hardly possible. But a flat or hollowed sheet
of *lead*, cast and hammered, to bake or fry on, was perfectly
easy, and Hofmann* reports such a lead baking sheet was
found. For lead-bronze hollow-ware they further refined the
shape and surface of round wares by machining them on a
lathe, like a potter's wheel, to get both better appearance and
a smoother surface that could be polished and oiled to reduce the uptake of copper (and of lead). Or they could have
used expensive tin.

Plautus in the second century B.C.[21] told of a banquet
served in *vasis stagneis*, probably pewter, lead-tin, an alloy
much harder and safer than pure lead.

A good examination of a different ancient ware, probably part of a pail, from a river Alpheus in Greece, of unknown date, was performed by Prof. E. R. Caley.[22] Its base

22. E. R. Caley: Chemical Examination of an Ancient Sheet of Metal;
   Ohio Jol. of Sci., 52:161-4, 1952. The triple alloyed coating was
   especially resistant to corrosion, Prof. Caley tells me.

was copper, and it had been coated both inside and out by plunging it into a molten alloy of about one-half copper, one-third tin, and one-sixth lead, which gave the vessel a whitish color. The base had been previously hammered onto a mold, to impart a *repoussé* design of considerable artistic merit; so the vessel must have held the food of well-to-do people. Pliny* (XIV:25-29) speaks of some such plating which shone like silver, and might have contained some. Even today there is sometimes objection to the little lead that comes from our silverplate.

Warnings of Lead's Danger

Some suspicion of the danger from hot lead in contact with acidic juices occurred to some ancient writers. Dioscorides* (V.9) said that corrected wine was "most hurtful to the nerves." Three times he speaks of wines that are constipating (V:10,11). And elsewhere, while recommending various lead medicines for external use, including the eyes, he recalled that internally lead is poison. Pliny* (XIV:21) said that wines like *oxymel* are condemned by Themison, "a very high authority," and do seem a *tour de force*, unnatural. In his following section, Pliny cited a wine of Arcadia that produced fertility in women and madness in men, whereas in another district of Greece a wine was reported to prevent child-bearing even if the women only ate the grapes, which yet tasted like others; in Thasos there was one wine that banished sleep, and another that brought abortion (XIV:19), and in Lycia a wine that constipated. All these are traits of lead poisoning, except fertility in women, which is obviously only a contrast with barrenness, likely connected with two differently made wines.

Pliny* wrote, after describing one of these leading procedures, "All these particulars show how successfully human intellect has pried into every secret" (15:21). And yet just before this passage Pliny had expressed doubt about the safety of artificial wines. Elsewhere he said he had not given much study to lead, for fear of wasting time.

Few passages in ancient literature indicate knowledge or

even suspicion of poisoning from mere *contact* of lead with acidic food (not water). One or two occur in Columella's* sixteen pages on viniculture. Apparently someone sometime had perceived that cooking acidic food in lead led to dysentery. For in XII:42 he gives a Greek recipe for a remedy against dysentery, the painful, often bloody constipative disorder which is typical of acute lead poisoning. To cure it he says to boil down raisin must in a new earthenware pot, or in one of tin *(stagneum)*, mix in quinces and pomegranates, and store it in new earthenware. The peculiar inclusion of two words of Greek in this section makes one suspect that it might be a later, Byzantine addition, altho the numbering of the sections is continuous.

One or two other hints of ancient awareness can be found in Soyer's* rare but useful *Pantropheon*, a history of cooking. It never indexes lead, but constantly cites the ancient authors, illustrates cooking wares, and says (about his page 263) that the richest had silver saucepans *(patinae)* as well as silver dishes; and he mentions silver plating. He also tells of preserving grapes for a year in rainwater (doubtless in a lead-lined cistern) which were then boiled down to one-third.

Some thot that the harm in sophisticated wines came from sweetness. In this they were not far misled. But we may reject a passage in the late writer Cassianus Bassus,[23] that ascribed to Democritos a recommendation to put in *sandyx* (red lead, minium, Pb_3O_4) to keep wine from going sour. For our oldest text of Cassianus comes from fifteen centuries later than Democritos, from a time when such practices of deliberate leading had come into use. The ancients knew lead and its salts to be poisonous if taken internally, tho they would use them externally, hardly ever fearing mere contact. Yet as one exception, Pliny* (34:52) says that the slag *(spodium)* of lead was sometimes ground up, sifted, and the powder put into aromatic, spiced wine.

Concerning the famous Falernian wine, the only one that would burn, Pliny* said (23:1) that when drunk tepid it "closes the belly, and some have thought that it dulls the vision and helps neither nerves nor bladder." And he said that wines from his home region, Pompeii, produced a long-lasting headache. All are symptoms of lead poison.

Serving Wine to the Wealthy

For a final touch of mis-led perfection, in cold weather in their unheated mansions, the wine and fruit drinks were warmed before serving in an ornamental heater of bronze, of course with lead where it mattered. (See Plate 8 on page 71.)

Wine was almost never drunk neat, but normally diluted with water. Straight wine was considered the drink of drunkards and barbarians. At a banquet the toastmaster would set the dilution rate, commonly to one-half, sometimes more. This would diminish the leading, even if the water had a little lead in it too.

Souring Vintage Wine

Roman vintners were well aware of the tendency of wine to go sour, so they had various ways to check on this threat. One was to suspend a strip of copper, lead, or tin in the air space at the top of an amphora, for forty days, to see if it would become powdery from the acidic vapor rising from souring wine. Some of the powder might fall into the wine. But this was the least important of the many ways that lead got into vintage wines. And so was another test Pliny* tells of: dipping a piece of lead into perhaps souring wine, to see if the lead changed color.[24]

Analyzing the Vintage Wines

A few ancient vintage wines have been *preserved to the present day* in certain amphoras, or where a glass bottle of wine was buried with its owner, and these have been analyzed for other substances, but not for lead. It should be possible for the right person to obtain small specimens of these wines, and perhaps of their drinker's bones, have them assayed for lead, and correlate the lead percentage with many other indications about the ancient user's wealth, age, sex, medical history, etc. One could thus manywise improve our knowledge of ancient leading and health, as we have sought to do in our book. Ten articles describing such ancient wines preserved to modern times are listed in Note 25. However, we have had wine *dust* from inside ancient amphoras analyzed and found lead in them, as reported in Appendix B, on page 201.

Grape Syrup

An important element of the Roman upper class diet was grape syrup, for sweetening drinks or other foods. It is still used in Turkey, Portugal, and other countries, including our own, where it is called grape concentrate and is an ingredient of commercial jams and jellies, of course without leading. But ancient grape syrup was sheer slow poison, made as described in Columella* (XII:19) and everywhere else. The ancient method of making it is depicted in Plates 16 and 18 on pages 77 and 78.

It was done by boiling down must (grape juice) in a leaden (or possibly lead-plated) pot, with constant stirring by a brush of twigs or fennel, to prevent any syrup from baking onto some spot and thus melting a hole thru a solid lead pot. The scraping must have enhanced the lead absorption.

This poisoned syrup was the Romans' favorite source for sweetening foods, and was sometimes used to keep wine from souring. Otherwise there was no sweetener save some other fruits cooked or preserved in the same leaded manner, and honey, which they also leaded sometimes (cf. *oxymel* below). Of course, honey must have been scarce and only for the well-to-do. After the third century A.D. the Romans imported a little sugar from India or Mesopotamia, but it must have been scarce and costly from its long transportation.

All folks have a great taste for sweeteners, as proved by the American economic consumption of refined sugar, 45 kg per year, 125 g per day, per capita in 1972, tho these figures, to be sure, are somewhat greater than those for our *dietary* consumption. Yet we have many other sources of sweeteners too, including fruits, honey, and artificial sweeteners.

Grape syrup of the ancients was *must*, boiled down to two-thirds, one-half, or one-third, and called variously *sapa*, *caroenum*, *carenum*, *defrutum* (for *defervitum*, "boiled down"), or sometimes by its Greek names *sireion*, *siracum*, or *hepsema*, according to the degree of boiling. The names varied somewhat, so we shall call them all grape syrup. References to such syrup are incessant in the ancient literature, and the recipes repeatedly involved lead in their making. Pliny* said (14:27): "Leaden and not bronze pots should be used." Cato* (105 and 122), Columella* (12:19, 20), and Palladius (X 3 Oct., 18) specify lead. Cato* (24) said to put a thirtieth part of grape syrup in every kind of artificial wine. Some other fruit of course could furnish some sweetness, especially dates and figs. And vairous fruits were preserved with grape syrup. When any acidic food was cooked, there stood always the old saturnine specter. Kobert* (p. 109) says all piquant sauces contained *defrutum*, and that most invertebrate and fish foods were preserved in it.

Duplicating Grape Syrup

Hofmann* performed an experiment to see how much lead would be introduced into grape syrup by the ancient procedures. A lead plate was put into white must which was then boiled down to one-half, as recommended by Pliny, except that it was not once stirred nor scraped, thus much reducing the leading. The surface of lead was 348 sq. cm., and the volume of the must 0.6 liter. After the boiling down to half the syrup held 237 mg. of lead per liter, a little of which had come from leaden parts still used in the Styrian winepress in 1884. Such a grape syrup (or lead syrup) was bad enough to sicken a man most severely by long consumption of one tablespoonful a day. A student of Prof. Clair C. Patterson, attempting to duplicate the Roman grape syrup, got 1000 ppm. lead.

According to a recent authoritative report "In evaluating the data from a number of studies of daily intake from air, food and water, it has been estimated that 300 micrograms of elemental lead should be the maximum daily permissible intake from all sources for children. It was the opinion of the committee which provided these data that if lead intakes exceed these limits, then the body can no longer effectively excrete the surplus lead, and accumulation with subsequent damage will occur."[26]

This proposed maximum permissible level of 300 micrograms is for children, who are considerably more vulnerable to lead poisoning then adults. Hence, a comparable adult level would be several times higher. But the Roman rate of lead ingestion was more than 700 times as great as that considered tolerable for American children in the 1970's. (The reader should remember that the American figures are in micrograms, millionths of a gram, whereas the Roman figures are in milligrams, thousandths of a gram.)

When we consider the apparent extent of lead poisoning in the Roman upper and middle classes, the wonder is not that this "silent epidemic" destroyed the brains of the greatest empire the world had known, but rather that it took so many centuries to finish them.

Fancier Drinks the Rich Fancied

The richer Romans had a number of other alcoholic drinks, first Mead, which they called by its Greek name *hydromel(i)*, water-honey, or sometimes *aqua mulsa*, or *melitites*.[27] It was made from honey and water, and Pliny said it was made from rainwater either kept five years or boiled down three times, evidently to let in lead. In 31:6 he said this mead was given to invalids craving wine, since it was weaker.

At a later date Cassianus Bassus[28] described *hydromel* as a mixture of apple-pulp with old rainwater, but said a better kind was cider mixed with honey and rainwater and boiled. Kobert* recalled[29] an ancient statement that *hydromel* cold was an aperient, loosening the bowels, but when hot (presumably cooked) it was anti-diarrhetic. These opposite effects of the cooked and uncooked varieties were undoubtedly due to lead, Kobert said, since one of the most obvious effects of this metal is to induce costiveness, constipation.[30]

Oxymel, "sharp honey," was a mixture of vinegar, honey and wine, and placed in the sun to age. The Romans who could afford it liked to drink it warmed, which would doubtless introduce more lead from the pot. Pliny* (14:21) would add salt to it, and boil it ten times; but we have cited his suspicion of it. Dioscorides* (5:22) gave a recipe for *oxymel*, including boiling it ten times, and named various diseases he thot it helped.

Mulsum, wine-honey, also called by its Greek name *oenomeli*, was especially enjoyed by the Romans for a first course, Pliny* and Hofmann said.[31] It figures in many of the recipes of Apicius'* cookbook. Four or five kg. of honey were mixed with nine liters of must, or of old wine. Columella said to make it by mixing ten pounds of honey (without wax) with three gallons of must, or old old wine. And Cassianus called for rainwater. Pliny* says it was boiled in a copper kettle (pretty surely involving lead).

Passum was a wine made from raisins or figs, which figures in 32 of Apicius' 478 major recipes. Columella* (XII: 39) said some people make it from old rainwater boiled down to one-third (two obvious means for getting lead). Athenaeus* following Polybius said that women might drink it, tho denied wine. Remark[32] says it was a drink for common people, citing Martial XII:124.

Some non-alcoholic beverages were also made from various fruit juices mixed with honey and vinegar, then boiled down to the consistency of honey. Of course the fruit acids, vinegar, heat, and lead would form the usual fateful combination. A myrtle or a quince drink *(Myrtites* or *Kydonites)* may have been among the worst, since Hofmann* says they were boiled down in a small leaden or bronze kettle.

Preserved fruits, preserved by cooking in lead, were another way for the wealthier class to please the palate and poison the diet, since they lacked the modern technique of sterilization by heat and then sealing hermetically. We read in Apicius* (I:12) how to preserve quinces in grape syrup boiled down to one-third, and likewise blackberries and olives. Kobert* (109) says that plums, cherries, apples, pears, peaches, quinces, etc. were prepared as today, and sweetened with grape syrup and cooked in lead. Such fruits would reach non-wine-drinkers.

Kinds of Water?

The ancient writers sometimes speak of different kinds of water, and what kind would serve best. Columella* (12:39) liked the recipe of the Carthaginian Mago for making *passum* by watering raisins and boiling the mixture down to a third; he points out that some people liked to use rainwater (doubtless drawn from a lead-lined cistern). Pliny* too specifies rainwater, altho he acknowledges in 31:21 that medical men say cistern water is harsh and bad for the bowels and throat, and is full of slime. Yet still he writes (14:20) that for making mead (honey-water) one should use rainwater five years old, "or some use fresh rainwater boiled three times." Any high school chemist will tell you that rainwater preserved no matter how long, or boiled any number of times, remains nothing but pure H_2O. But the Romans knew otherwise. For they would have kept the water in a cistern lined with lead, which the rainwater would take up, being neutral, or the more so if it had been acidulated by leaves washed off the roof and down the lead drainpipe. Also the rainwater boiled would have been boiled in some kind of leaded pot.

The Low-Grade Wines of the Lowly, but with Less Lead

How the wines for the slaves and other workers were made, and presumably for the poor in general, is told, e.g., by Pliny* (XIV:12), who speaks of three kinds of *lora*, also called *vappa*, for them. One kind was made from the second squeezing of the grape skins, after watering and soaking them. A second kind, habitual with the Greeks, would add a third as much water as the must previously pressed out, and then boiled down to one-third this watered pressing, thereby doubtless leading it. The third kind, *faecatum*, was pressed out from the wine lees. None of these three would keep more than a year. The two Roman kinds, the first and third, would have no sources of lead but the winepress and a much used leaden strainer *(colum)*, while the second, leaded kind was that of the Greeks. All were left in the great fermenting vat, *dolium,* to make *vinum doliare* or *de cupa,* not racked off into amphoras; and none would keep for more than a year, Pliny said. All three of these wines for the poor we shall call *vat wines.* They apparently served most of the poor, and were almost free from lead. Other ancient writers indicated similarly.

Yet it seems likely that the poor also got a good deal of leaded wine that had been intended for the rich, but which had gone sour, and hence would be sold cheap, or given to slaves. For the ancient viniculturists often speak of wine souring. This might well have happened often because it had not been sufficiently leaded. Likewise *vinegar,* an important factor in the poor and military diets, might have been made, one would think, from such spoiled vintage wine, which yet had some lead in it. But more likely from wine which had gone sour because it was not leaded.

On the whole the poor had the advantage that their wine was much less leaded (since the rich might put lead into their wine in a dozen ways, above all by boiling it in lead, and by adding grape syrup). But likely the poors' greatest escape from lead was that they had less wine, and still less of fancy alcoholic drinks, and of grape syrup. Also poor women got much less than their men, since nothing is said about wine for them. And it is especially in women that lead poisoning is disastrous for offspring.

Still the poor, including slaves, got considerable lead too, it will appear from their bones, in our Chapter 8. This lead would come from the very dangerous lead trades, and probably from leaden, pewter or lead-lined cooking vessels, and, as we said, from wine intended for the well-to-do, which had spoiled.

Probably the least poisoned people would be poor peasants living in remote or mountainous areas, who could afford little wine, grape syrup or preserved fruits, but had wood fuel cheap, so that they cooked and stored food cheaply enough in clay pots locally fired, rather than in metal vessels bought from distant cities.

Olives and Olive Oil

Olives and their oil were important parts of the upper class diet, and would commonly add some lead, according to the procedures reported. Pliny* (XV:6), citing Cato,* said the best olives were steeped in grape syrup. And some were boiled. Also leaden cauldrons should be used, he said, since copper spoils the oil. The oil was abundantly used, as we said, for oiling bronze pots, against copper poisoning. Columella* (XII:50) likewise says to preserve olives in grape syrup, and in vinegar. Olives were pressed in presses like those described for wine, having lead tanks, pipes and strainers. But much of the olive oil was burnt in lamps. Still its lead could be breathed, which is worse than eating it.

Comparative Prices

Some comparative prices may be of interest, from 301 A.D. when Diocletian imposed on the Empire his comprehensive system of price controls. Grape syrup had its price fixed at 160 denarii for a gallon (about 4 liters). The best honey cost 320 denarii the gallon, but Phoenician date honey could be purchased for 64. Some of the other prices for food and drink were: ordinary wine 64 denarii the gallon, first-class wine 192, olive oil 96, and beer 32. An egg or an oyster cost 1 denarius, a dormouse 4, and mutton or goat meat about 5.4 denarii per kilogram.

Summarizing the Food of the Rich and Poor

We should say that the wines of the wealthy and other alcoholic drinks, including some prescribed as medicines, were always somewhat leaded, and often heavily, while those of the poor averaged much less poisonous. And the poor had some beer instead of wine, and beer was probably lead free.

Also the *women* of the poor apparently got much less wine than their men. And they do the child-bearing and suckling in which lead matters most.

1.   Pliny,* Rackham trans., Loeb, XIV:ii, 8.
2.   Pliny,* XIV, xvii, 97.
3.   See the note on page 29.
4.   Pliny,* XIV, xiv, 89-91.
5.   See the note on page 30.
6.   W. E. H. Lecky: *History of European Morals from Augustus to Charlemagne*, 1869, I:96.
7.   See the note on page 30.
8.   Polybius: *Histories*, VI:2, said they could drink *passum vinum*.
9.   Propertius: *Elegies*, iv, 8. Quoted in Wm. Younger: *Gods, Men and Wine*, p. 181.
10. Martial, *Epistles*, III:77; v. 64, 14 1n3 110.
11. Ovid, quoted in Younger, *supra*, p. 215.
12. W. Ward Fowler: *Social Life at Rome in the Age of Cicero*, (Lon., MacMillan, 1965), pp. 39, 40.
13. *Oxford Classical Dictionary*, 2nd ed., 1970, article on Wine.
14. Suetonius: *The Deified Augustus*, II:42.
15. Jon & Julia Solomon: *Ancient Roman Feasts and Recipes*, adapted for modern cooking; 144 pp.; 1977, E. A. Seeman pub., Miami.
16. See the note on page 35.
17. See the note on page 35.
18. Pliny,* 34:49, end.
19. Works on Roman viniculture overlooking lead, 3 dissertations and a book:

     Orth, Ferd.; *Weinbau u. Weinbereitung der Römer*, 59 pp., 1902.

     Gustav Lehman: *De Vinis apud Romanos*, a gymnasium dissertation in 1872, 18 pp.

     Luigi Manzi's doctoral dissertation in Italy in 1883 on ancient Roman wines, 130 pp.

     Andrea Bacci: *De Naturali Vinorum Historia*, 1596, 370 pp., a prodigious history of wines.
20. Apicius,* p. 34 and its editors' commentary.
21. Kobert,* pp. 108 and 111.
22. See the note on page 39.
23. Hofmann,* p. 284 and its Note 2, citing Cassianus Bassus: *Geoponica*, VI:19.
24. Pliny,* 14:25.
25. Forbes, 1st ed., p. 101, from our footnote *16*, citing B. Bruyère' *Les Fouilles de Deir el Medineh*, 1937, p. 1097, incl. preserved jars of Egyptian grape syrup.

     Herb W. Allen: *History of Wine*, 1961; opposite p. 34 shows wine preserved at museum of Speyer, Germany.

     A. Marescalchi & G. Dalmasso: *Storia della Vite e del Vino*, 1931-

7; 3:317 illustrates the same.

R. Billiard: *La Vigne dans l'antiquité*, 1913, 560 pp.; p. 529 for the wine specimen from Aliscamps.

Ch. Anthon: *Greek & Roman Antiques*, p. 694.

Joh. Grüss: Ueber den ältesten Weinreste . . . auf deutschen Boden: *Forschungen u. Fortschritte*, Feb. 1939, pp. 103-5.

Berthelot: Analyse d'un vin antique, from Aliscamps: *Annales de Chimie et de Physique*, 5th ser., 12:413-8, 1877. Or in *Rev. Archeol.*, ser. 2, vol. I:392-6.

Chas. Seltman: *Wine in the Ancient World*, Lon., 1957.

Celi examined wine from the house of M. Cassius of Pompeii, according to L. Manzi's dissertation (see Note 19 above).

Ph. Diolé: *4000 Years under the Sea*, tr. by Hopkins, 1952.

26.   Jas. M. McCullough: *Environmental Health Effects of Lead: An analysis of the issues and Congressional actions.* (Revised). Lib. of Congress Congressional Research Service, TN 480 75-95 SP, March 15, 1975, p. 6.

27.   Pliny,* 14:11 and 14:25.

28.   Cassianus Bassus: *Geoponica*, 25, 37.

29.   Kobert,* pp. 108 and 111.

30.   Kobert,* pp. 104-5.

31.   Pliny,* 34, 49, end.

32.   Peter Remark: *Der Weinbau im Römerreiche*, 1927, 110 pp.; on *passum* cites Martial XIII:125. He was familiar with Hofmann's* discoveries on lead.

5

Other Ways to Get Lead

The Roman rich had many ways to get lead into their bodies, beside their perversity for putting it into their foods (discussed in our previous chapter), and into their drinking water (in our next chapter). They seemed as devoted to the saturnine metal as to its joint product silver, or to the enlargement of their empire. The clever class found many ways to use this cheap and handy metal, so readily fashioned, thruout their homes and environment.

Pigments

The pigments the ancients favored were derived from both vegetal and mineral substances; but the former need not concern us, nor the non-poisonous minerals. Bright colors were favored, as they tend to be in countries of bright sunshine. Colors we might call garish in New York or London were popular in the homes of those who could afford such luxuries. Even their statues, in sunny courtyards, were usually painted. A bright red, familiar to us from the fine mansions of Pompeii and Herculaneum, was a very popular wall paint, and was doubtless used in the rich homes of Rome and elsewhere. (See Plate 19 on page 79, showing a wall painting in a home in Pompeii, using much red paint.) Red lead, minium, made a favorite paint. Its use for the red ink in medieval manuscripts has given us the word miniature. Outdoors sun and rain would change it to red-brown, as on our steel bridges and frieght cars today. Its source was litharge (PbO), a yellowish-red ore, which was changed to minium (Pb_3O_4) by heating it in air. This red minium may have had a

52

sacred meaning. It was used to paint the face of the image of Jove, as well as the bodies of conquering generals in their triumphal processions.

But there were other red paints too. One was based on cinnabar, an ore of mercury, which would be harmless if it were pure mercuric sulfide, but which often contains droplets of pure mercury, very poisonous, by air or mouth. Another and cheaper red was based on hematite (Fe_2O_3), a harmless iron oxide.

Whatever the paint, the wealthy inhabitants of the Empire were bound to pick up some, especially from its falling to the floor, whence to toddlers' hands and mouths. Leaden dust might also be kicked into the air, especially the lower air breathed by little folks. Numerous sad examples are at hand from recent times, from the children of lead-working fathers who brot home the saturnine stuff on their clothes, to tenement dwellers whose old homes had also been painted with lead-based paints, which for the last generation have been banned from interior use.

Litharge (PbO) also made a yellow pigment, with, of course, a different preparation. And another yellow paint was lead antimonate, $Pb_3(SbO_4)_2$. A white pigment was ceruse, $PbCO_3$,[1] which also makes white lead, approximately $2PbCO_3 \cdot Pb(OH)_2$. And white lead mixed with lead acetate and heated yielded a gray paint. Thus we have six lead compounds, their greatest use being for coloring walls.

For such painting, the techniques of both dry and true fresco were used. Dry fresco is painting with a tempera technique[2] on a dry prepared wall, so that the pigment becomes part of the wall. Both types of fresco would naturally in time drop dust in the areas involved, leaden dust, if the paint were leaded. Flakes would also drop occasionally, one would think, or might be plucked from the wall and eaten by children, if pica, the habit of eating strange objects, existed then

2.   The tempera technique is a method of mixing dry, powdered pigment with a medium such as water or egg white, and applying it with a brush to a previously prepared surface.

as today in our slums, altho it is fostered by a sense of deprivation.

One would think that all such painting would concern only the rich, and the artisans who prepared it, and that the poor and the slaves would be lucky to have whitewash, or bare plaster. Yet Friedländer[3] said that Roman art was "subserving all needs and tastes, the highest and the lowest" and that it even beautified the poor slave's cell, and covered the walls of taverns and brothels. Yet it is self-evident that the rich not only commissioned superior paintings, but had a large number of them. Of the 2,500 paintings preserved for us at Pompeii, thanks to Vesuvius (more than are extant from all the rest of the classical world), no less than 192 were found in one house, that of the Vettii. Art painting was done on a mass production basis, thru guilds. But the rich had more means than the poor to keep their floors clean.

The painter himself was also in danger. The emperors Nero, Trajan, Hadrian, Marcus Aurelius, Elagabalus, Valentinian, and Alexander Severus were all painters.[4] With lead paints this is a dangerous occupation, if, as likely, they ground their paints in mortars and mixed them on their pallets, as did Francisco Goya. That great Spanish painter (1746-1828), who had been thot to be syphilitic, who suffered a great mental crisis, and who lost children in rapid succession, has been diagnosed by the modern physician Niederland[5] as suffering from lead poisoning. He mixed his own paints, largely lead-based, and worked tremendously. Fetal deaths are one symptom of paternal plumbism.

Ramazzini[6] in his 1713 book on the *Diseases of Workers* commented on the ill health of painters, including "those of great fame." Even at that date he concluded that ninety to one hundred percent of all plumbism from handling white paints went undetected. In Roman times perhaps superior Greek slaves and upper class artists were especially affected and afflicted.

Cosmetics

Cosmetics were especially harmful when leaden, because

they affected *women*, the child-bearers and the sucklers and holders of infants. And of course cosmetics were used only by the upper and middle classes, not by the poor; so they were aristocidal.

Ceruse, the previously mentioned combination of the carbonate and hydroxide of lead, was the favorite white cosmetic in ancient times. It was used as a face powder, and sometimes for the hair, or to cover blemishes. In Europe ceruse continued in occasional use into the eighteenth century; in Oman it continues to modern times. Its somewhat variable composition has been discussed by Stevenson[1] and others; but in any case it was leaden, and the ancients seem to have had no idea of harm from using it externally on sores and wounds and to cover blemishes, even tho they knew it was poison if taken internally. Whether it or any form of lead can be absorbed by rubbing into intact skin is disputed. But there can be no question that the use of these cosmetics would lead to some of them getting into the eyes or mouth, or worse, being inhaled by the woman or her nursing baby. Among Japanese in Manchuria in 1925 ceruse was the fourth greatest cause of infant mortality, and it was still common in Japan in 1933.[7] Ovid recommended this ceruse in his pleasant poetry,[8] and Martial and Athenaeus* speak of it. Xenophon[9] presents a man Isomachus urging his young wife against using it, as well as minium (lead) rouge; he argues with her for a page or more against them, but never mentions any reason of health. The fine ladies of Greece were so fond of ceruse (tho sunlight turned it yellow) that they were sometimes entombed with a covered container (a *pyxis)* of it beside them. Plate 13 on page 75 shows such a Corinthian container with its pretty poison.[10]

Minium rouge on the lips would be sure to be swallowed. On the forehead it is still used in India. But sometimes the ancients substituted harmless red ocher, an iron ore. The dark lead ore galena (PbS), or poisonous antimony, are both still used in Egypt and Pakistan, to darken the eyelids and eyebrows.[11]

Aside from professional courtesans and prostitutes, the groups whose women were most exposed to this type of lead

poisoning in Greece and Rome were the rich, the successful,
the eminent. Women of the upper classes could afford to
beautify themselves with cosmetics; but the impact was
aristocidal.

Contraception and Abortion

The Greco-Roman acceptance and over-use of birth
control (considered more fully in Chapter 10), was a contrib-
utory cause in the reproductive failure of the upper class. In
Chapter 3 we cited the methods of Aristotle and Soranus,
which prescribed lead ointments for contraception and leaded
drinks for oral contraception and abortion. From modern
clinical studies we know that use of lead preparations in vaginal douches can cause lead poisoning. The ointments recommended by Aristotle and Soranus were probably likewise
dangerous.

What classes used these lead contraceptives and aborti-
facients? Members of all ranks attempted birth control, but
the poor, without access to trained physicians, doubtless relied more on the useless magical procedures. The upper classes were better informed; they often used lead products and
achieved the desired result, tho sometimes sterilizing themselves in the process. Courtesans and prostitutes would
necessarily be skilled in birth control.

Other Medical Uses

That lead sulfide and litharge were used to cicatrize
wounds has been told in Chapter 3. They would indeed help
heal the wound, yet they would also impart lead.

Since Greek and Roman physicians were aware of the
poisonous nature of lead salts, they seldom knowingly recommended that they be eaten or drunk. An exception was
Alexander of Tralles, a Greek physician of the sixth century
B.C., who thot that lead pills helped cure hardened feces.[12]

The main danger from these medical practices was that
in bringing lead or its compounds into direct contact with
open wounds, lesions, and ulcers, and into the vaginal tract

and rectum, they invited poisoning of the bloodstream and the genito-urinary system.

Toys

The impact of lead on patrician life began early; it first threatened conception, then successful pregnancy, and later infant survival, especially thru cosmetics, paints, and even the toys given Roman children. This latter menace operated mostly against the rich, save for lead workers. For toys cost money.[13]

Children were not considered important people, so little is to be found on the tykes' toys in the surviving literature. What we now know of them is the result of modern archeology.

It appears that dolls were made of wax or of unglazed terra cotta. Such things as spindles, tops, and other toys might be wooden, or could be of leaden material, and there would be the danger. Plate 14 on page 76 shows an ancient leaden wheel, about ten cm. in diameter, that Gilfillan photographed in the Museum of Reggio, Calabria.

Any toys of lead would be a threat to children thru handling or mouthing. We must remember that children are much more susceptible to lead than adults, and that only families of some means could provide such toys. The leaden toys were probably unpainted, but they might possibly have been painted with minium, red lead. So every touch might spell poison.

Perhaps the worst toys were the *crepundia*, "rattling things" (see Plate 15 on page 76),[14] small trinkets hung on a string around a child's neck, for his amusement and to ward off witchcraft. These were of many substances, but usually metal. If the parents were among the wealthiest patricians in the Empire, the *crepundia* could possibly have been made of precious metals, or bronze, brass, or pewter. But another metal would be more usual—simple lead—the commonest and cheapest metal in the ancient world. Moreover, *crepundia* were given only to the offspring of freeborn Romans, thus saving the poorest classes from this exposure to lead.

Crepundia were to keep a child quiet. One of the periods when a child is most distressed is when teething. And the *crepundia* might have been used to let a child teethe on them. The soft metal need present no sharp edges. So the children of the upper class could have begun their lifelong lead poisoning early, literally by cutting their teeth on it.

Lead-Glazed Art Pottery

Glazes for pottery had two important uses. They served to make ancient porous clayware (like our terra cotta, not at all like our chinaware) impenetrable to liquids that would foul it. And they provided an esthetically pleasing coating that covered blemishes and could carry rich decoration, altho with only a few colors. The unglazed earthenware was used for most purposes, but where beauty was desired and could be paid for, a lead glaze was added.

The Egyptians had for 2,000 years used a harmless and unimportant silicious lead glaze; and about 100 B.C. Mesopotamians put lead glazes on tiles and bricks, but not on pottery. The Greeks used alkaline black and a few other colors in glazed ware. But it was only around the beginning of the Christian era that dangerous, lustrous, lead-glazed ware became common thruout the Roman world, especially for cups, bowls, and pitchers in which acidic food might stand. Plate 1 on page 67 is an example; a beaker 15.3 cm. high, Alexandrian, of about 10 A.D.[15] But the skeleton on it is ironic only to us. To the ancients it signified "Eat, drink, and be merry, for tomorrow we die," further expressed in the inscription KTO XPO (buy and consume). Another expression of this thot is the skeleton mosaic from Pompeii in Plate 21 on page 81.

Proper firing was undoubtedly the most difficult and often defective step. After the original firing, the baked ware had to be painted, glazed, and then again fired for a long time and at temperatures of over 1000°C.[16] Roman kilns could reach these temperatures, but they were hard to maintain. Fuel was expensive because of competing uses, dwindling forests, and costly land transportation, from the inefficient traction afforded by the poor design of the ancient harness, and lack of horseshoes. Nor was there any good way for the buyer or the maker to judge the firing of the product. A vessel could look properly fired even if the kiln had not reached the required temperature, or maintained it long enough. Without a pyrometer, there was no good way to control or assess quality.

Thus, most glazed Roman pottery (like some today from Mexico and China, or from the kilns of American amateur potters) was inadequately fired. In Germany in 1893, 65 percent of glazed ware submitted to a research institute was judged faulty. In Livonia, 56 percent of such pottery gave up lead on the first cooking of vinegar.[17]

For most foods, Roman glazed pottery was reasonably safe as well as attractive. But for holding the acidic drinks the upper classes enjoyed, it was dangerous. And the Romans seemed to use glaze most for pitchers, vases, and cups, where lengthy standing would be likely for the mixing, temporary storage, and serving of beverages. Since the favorite drinks of the upper class derived from fermented or unfermented fruits and were hence acidic, they interacted with the glaze to give their wealthy users another dose of lead.

But the plebeians were no doubt less affected, as the result of a less acidic diet, and of unglazed pottery, simple terra cotta, made anywhere by a single, moderate firing.

Lead glaze had two dangers, the greater being that of giving up lead by contact, especially long and/or hot contact with any acidic food. But in addition another danger was the seemingly trivial act of scratching a plate. Some of the scratched-off powder could be swallowed, and the stomach's hydrochloric acid would dissolve it. And this could occur even if the ware had been properly fired.

Writing Implements

Writing in Rome was as necessary as today for running a civilization. So everyone who needed to could read and write. But the poor rarely needed to. Almost all the slaves who were not household servants were illiterate, as were the bulk of the freeborn rural poor. As for the Roman legions, we have Vegetius' fourth century manual of military training, in which he points out that such army jobs as keeping payroll rosters, require *litterati milites.* So we can infer that the bare literacy required for keeping records was beyond the average Roman soldier.

For paper the Romans used pages or rolls of papyrus, on which they wrote with harmless inks. We are not concerned with these, but rather with leaden equipment for writing, especially what was handled by children. The implements most often mentioned for schools were tablets of lead, so soft one could even write on them with a fingernail. (These tablets could also be wood, covered with wax and marked with a stylus of metal or bone.) But lead was cheap and could make a true "lead" pencil to write on papyrus paper. If either the tablet or the pencil were of lead, this might be rubbed onto the hands and thence carried to the mouth, or the stylus or pencil might be touched to the lips. While lead absorption from one of these acts would be minuscule, many contacts might add up to a serious threat to someone doing much writing, or to any schoolchild.

Miscellaneous Uses of Lead

Some dysgenically questionable or dangerous uses of lead included coins in Egypt and Gaul, all kinds of tickets, medals of Christian devotion, votive offerings at shrines, dangerous clamps to mend cracked amphoras or *dolia* (vats—Plate 4 on page 89), lead hoops for wine barrels, nesting of iron or bronze clamps, joint tighteners in furniture, lead anchors, sheathing to protect the whole hull of a ship from the shipworm *(teredo),* plummets, scourges, sewer pipes, and especially roofs, drain pipes, cisterns, baths, tanks, pails, and decorative drinking cups (Plate 12 on page 73). All uses for containing potable water were very dangerous, unless the water was hard or the exposure very brief, as we shall explain in our next chapter. Carcopino* is a good source.

The industries for making all these leaden things were very unhealthy for the artisans, especially when the lead was melted, or soldered, and worst of all, in its mining and smelting. So the lower class were much affected and afflicted by most of these uses of lead, tho less on the whole than the rich, since only a fraction of the poor were lead workers or part of their families.

1.   Stevenson,* Appendix A, pp. 404-410; also his On the Meaning of the Words Cerussa and Psimithium, *Jol. of Med. & Allied Sci.*, 10:109-11, 1955.
2.   See the note on page 53.
3.   Ludwig Friedländer: *Roman Life and Manners under the Early Empire:* Lon., 1908-13, 3 vols., 2:268. One may see also Amedeo Maiuri: *Roman Painting*, Geneva, Skira, for its reproductions, pp. 51-61; or Jean Mercadé, Geneva, Nagel, pp. 60, 61.
4.   Friedländer, supra, 2:327-8.
5.   W. G. Niederland: Goya's Illness: a Case of Lead Encephalopathy? *N. Y. State Jol. of Med.*, Feb. 1, 1972, pp. 413-9.
6.   B. Ramazzini: *Diseases of Workers*, 1964, tr. from *De Morbis Artificum*, 1713.
7.   T. S. Rodgers & Peck & Jupe: Lead Poisoning in Children; *Lancet*, 2:129, 1934. Also T. Suzuki and J. Kaneko: Serous Meningitis in Infants, caused by lead poisoning from white powders: *Jol. Oriental Medicine*, 9:55-66, 1925.
8.   Ovid: *Remedia Amoris*, or *De Medicamine Faciei*, line 73. Cf. also Martial: *Epigrams*, I:72-5.
9.   Xenophon: *OEconomicus*, X:5.
10.   Leslie Shear, in *Classical Studies Presented to Edw. Capps*, 1949, Princeton, pp. 314-7, fig. 10 used.
11.   H. A. Warley & Blackledge & O'Forman: Lead Poisoning from Eye Cosmetics: *British Med. Jol.*, 1:117 ff., 1968.
12.   Alexander von Tralles: *Original-Text und Uebersetzung*, 1879, II: 362.
13.   J. P. V. D. Balsdon: *Life and Liesure in Ancient Rome*, N.Y., McGraw-Hill, or Lon., Bodley Head, 1969, p. 91.
14.   Harold W. Johnston: *Private Life of the Romans*, 1903, 344 pp., well illus., p. 69, whence our Plate 15.
15.   Gaetano Ballardini: *L'Eredità Ceramistica dell' Antico Mondo Romano:* 1964, 8°, 308 pp; pp. 98, 99 for the lead beaker. It is in the Staatlicher Museen Preussischer Kulturbesitz, DI W. Berlin 19.
16.   C. W. Parmelee: *Ceramic Glazes*, 1948, pp. 22 and 27.
17.   Rosenblatt,* pp. 10, 11.

6

Lead from the Water Supply

The ancient Romans, and probably the Greeks before them, certainly took in much lead from their water supply, where the water was not hard. Hard water is calcareous from limestone and takes up little or no lead.[1] Usually the water was either neutral (e.g. rainwater) or acidic from decaying vegetation or volcanic soil. There was a town near Naples, ancient Puteoli (modern Pozzuoli), with a hot spring where Pausanias[2] said the acidic water would perforate a pipe in a few years. The water evidently contained sulfurous acid. Of the aqueducts of Rome, only some supplied hard, harmless water from limestone country. Athens' aqueduct water was hard, but its rainwater was not. The Mediterranean region has various volcanic regions producing acidic or neutral water.

Lead was not merely the ancients' only cheap metal (aside from iron, which was unusable for water supply then), but lead was also the only cheap metal they could easily work. For they could not cast, truly weld, roll nor draw iron, nor easily hammer it thin. Moreover iron rusts. So they used lead for water pipes, roofs, drainpipes, and for the lining of cisterns and baths, with the special merit for baths that its metal would transmit heat much better than masonry or unreinforced cement. Also a leaden roof could be near flat, like ours of galvanized steel or cement, and could save scarce fuel for firing terra cotta. And when an aqueduct or urban distribution system had to carry water under pressure,

---

1.   Like the calcium in milk, the lime in hard water tends to prevent the take-up of lead from a container, because the calcium in lime is a related and rival element to lead.

because it had gone downhill faster than the very minimum, lead was desirable because it was strong and kept tight joints. The four aqueducts for Lyon in France used 10,000 tons of lead pipes to carry water under the Rhone.[3] But occasionally bored logs, or pottery, were used, and for terminals of the wealthy there was lead-bronze, probably for ostentation, as with silver. The incrustations of time however, might reduce lead take-up. Many of us have stumbled over lead pipes in the dirt sidewalks of Pompeii (Plate 12 on page 74), where the water was certainly acidic from sulfur and volcanic soil. Moreover many of the pipes there and often elsewhere were not cast, and therefore not cylindrical (see Plate 11 on page 74). Instead they had a tear-drop cross-section, composed of a curve and an angle, made by bending lengthwise a long strip of cast lead, and soldering the two edges together. This gave more lead surface per liter of flow than would a circular pipe. The fittings, the stops, were of lead or bronze, which also always contained lead.

We should poke further into those leaden cisterns. There the neutral rainwater would remain for months, from the winter thru the long, almost rainless Mediterranean summer, to the dog days and the vintage. (And we shall speak in Chapter 14 of the worsening of this climate.) In such a cistern, lead would be taken up by neutral rainwater, and more so if leaves had been washed down from the flat roof, making the water acidulous. Pliny* says, "As to cistern water, medical men assure us that owing to its harshness it is bad for the bowels and throat; and it is generally admitted that there is no kind of water that contains more slime or more numerous insects of disgusting nature" (31:21). Yet we observe in our fourth chapter the same ancient encyclopedist writing (14:20) that mead *(hydromel)* should be made from rainwater kept for five years, or else boiled down to one-third. Evidently he wanted lead for its sterilizing properties against souring, not knowing that it could also sterilize its drinkers. There would be no point in calling for such long stored or boiled-down rainwater unless the neutral water were meant to take up lead from its container. Cassianus Bassus[4] similarly said that mead is to be made from stale rainwater boiled down to a third, mentioning the staleness three times and the boiling twice. Columella,*[5] who called for leaden boiling pots seven times in four pages, twice asked for sea water kept for three years, presumably in a lead-lined cistern, and for boiling it down to a third. Again, after mentioning Mago's method for making raisin wine, he said to use old rainwater boiled down to one-third. There would again be no point in aging or boiling it down, unless to take up lead. Apicius'* mostly high-class cookbook (I:12) recommended preserving grapes in rainwater boiled down to one-third, and to give such water to the sick.

At last Aëtius,[6] a Greek physician of the sixth century A.D., condemned lead roofs as a cause of dysentery. A physician in Britain was warning people about similar lead-lined cisterns as late as 1820.[7] For such dangerous uses of lead with neutral or acidulous water lasted abundantly thru the Middle Ages and down to the last century, while minor cases are even to be found in our homes today,[8] especially in the soldering of copper or galvanized iron pipes by lead-tin, and sometimes in the use of a solid lead pipe to connect a house with the street main, for the sake of lead's flexibility. All are harmless if the water is hard.

Another frequent misuse of lead was for pails, in which soft water, milk, or other and more lead-taking liquids might be left standing for long hours. Doubtless there were tanks too, for still longer holding. (Plate 2 on page 68 gives a sample.) If pails[9] and tanks are rare in museums, it is because they have had little artistic, and considerable scrap value. Our familiar modern pail, made by cooperage ("the old oaken bucket"), was a northern invention that reached Rome only about the beginning of our era. So as we said, Diogenes never saw a tub, but found shelter under a broken pottery vat.

With water as with all the other uses of lead, the ancients had little idea of danger from mere contact with the

9.   When a pail or other leaden object was lost in a well, that would somewhat poison water not hard. So we have questioned the lead findings in our bones from wells.

saturnine metal. We shall cite the only protests we have been able to find. Vitruvius,[10] a civil engineer about 23 B.C., said that water from earthenware pipes is much wholesomer than from lead, because from that metal comes poisonous white lead, and we know the pallor and weakness of lead workers. Also the flavor of water from clay pipes is better, Vitruvius said, and even those who can load their tables with silverware use earthen vessels to preserve the flavor of water. (Perhaps he was thinking of the coolness from evaporation of water that had soaked thru an unglazed pottery vessel.) But Frontinus (ca. 98 A.D.)[11] in his 65-page work on the water supply of Rome, took lead pipes for granted in many places, especially for the final distribution of the water, and while always concerned about the water's quality, seems to consider this only a matter of clarity versus muddiness or foul ingredients. But the great physician Galen[12] (130-200 A.D.) echoed Vitruvius' warnings, for avoiding dysentery. Palladius[13] (371-95 A.D.) gave a like warning emphatically, yet proceeded to give the dimensions for the lead pipes. And the emperor Antoninus had a water pipe partly of silver. Aside from these five cases we find no sure indication that leaded water was ever feared. To be sure, the poet Horace[14] (ca. 20 B.C.) asked if city water bursting from a leaden pipe is purer than that which hurries murmuring down a stream; but he could easily have had other reasons beside the saturnine one for thinking country water healthier than that from the city supply.

The Class Angle?

Was there a dysgenic or class angle to the water supply? One would think that rich and poor drank the same water, at least in the cities served by an aqueduct and by lead pipe distribution of soft or acidic water. The eugenic or dysgenic angle is our main problem, for this book and for all humanity in the long run.

There doubtless was such an angle, but we cannot prove which way it slanted, in this matter of the water supply. As for the water drunk, we think it tended rather to liquidate the more intelligent people, in that all the leaden installations we have been talking about were probably commoner in cities than in the countryside. Certainly aqueducts and pipe distribution were. And brains, whether free or slave, must have tended, as today, to gravitate to the cities, especially the capitals. Modern statistics show tremendous differences in eminence between men from the city versus those from the countryside.[15] To be sure, the wealthiest of Rome often vacationed in country estates. In rural areas the rich and their retinues might well have a lead roof and cistern, but they would be likely to depend more on some nearby spring, stream, or well; and still more so would the scattered peasantry.

But on the other hand, those pipes, roofs, cisterns, tanks, and pails added up doubtless to the greatest category of the *use* of lead. And the work of fabricating and installing all of them was performed in deadly surroundings by *poor* men almost exclusively, even if we do not count here the slaves who died in the silver/lead mines, but only count the *plumbarii* who fabricated the saturnine metal and breathed in its pestilent fumes. *Tu plumbarie!* You plumber! You crazy lead-worker! This was a common term of reproach in ancient times, as we noted in Chapter 3.

1.   See the note on page 62.
2.   Pausanias: *Description of Greece*, II, 34.
3.   C. J. Singer et al., eds.: *History of Technology*, 2:671, 1956 ed., citing O. Stübinger: *die Römischen Wasserleitungen.*
4.   Cassianus Bassus: *Geoponica*, chapters 36, 38.
5.   At the start of his Chapter 19.
6.   Aëtius: *Tetrabiblos*, III:i:45.
7.   Accum, Fredk.: *Treatise on Adulterations*, 1820.
8.   Stöfen, D.: Health Dangers of Lead in Drinking Water: *Zts. Präventifmed*, 16:325-32, 1971. In English.
9.   See the note on page 64.
10.   Vitruvius: *De Architectura*, VIII, cap. vi, par. 10, 11.
11.   Frontinus: *The Aqueducts of Rome*, e.g., I:25 and II:112.
12.   Galen,* in Kuhn ed., Bk. 13, p. 45.
13.   Palladius: *De Re Rustica*, IX:11.
14.   Horace: *Epistles*, I:10, 28.
15.   S. S. Visher: Some Influences Affecting the Productivity of Leaders: *Eugenical News*, 35:57-60, 1950.

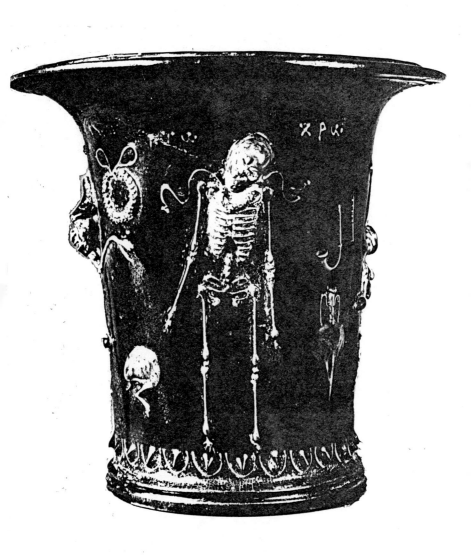

Plate 1. Alexandrian lead-glazed beaker of 10 A.D., 15 cm. high. The skeleton signified to the ancients, "Eat, drink and be merry, for tomorrow we die." (See the cover and page 58.)
Courtesy of the Statlicher Museen Preussicher Kulturbesitz, West Berlin.

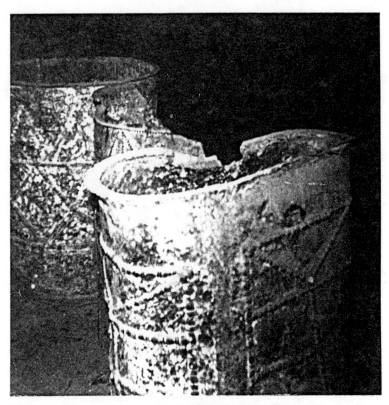

Plate 2. Lead tanks of artistic character, which the author photographed in the Museo Nazionale of Naples. (See pages 11 and 64.)

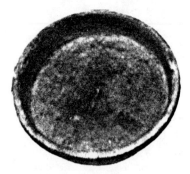

Plate 3. Roman pewter plate photographed by the author in the Museo Nazionale of Naples. (See page 12.)

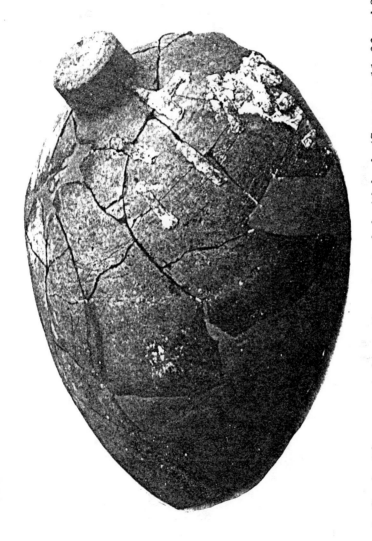

Plate 4. Greek *pithos*, ceramic fermenting vat, mended with lead. (See pages 11, 36 and 37.) Used with permission from R. L. Scranton; "The Pottery from the Pyramics," in *Hesperia*, 7:533-4, figure 5.

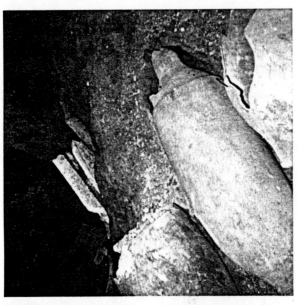

Plate 6. Ceramic amphoras recently excavated in Pompeii. The author received permission to take a sample of the dust from inside the center one and had it analyzed for lead. Photo by the author. (See pages 36 and 201.)

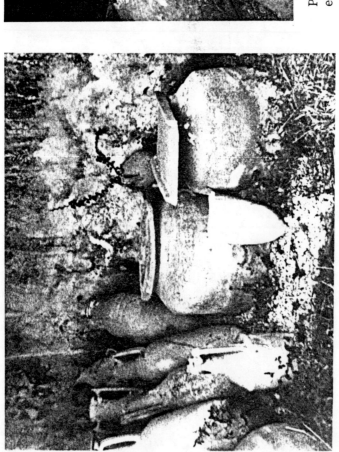

Plate 5. Ceramic amphoras and jars found in Pompeii. The amphoras stored wine. Photo by the author. (See page 36.)

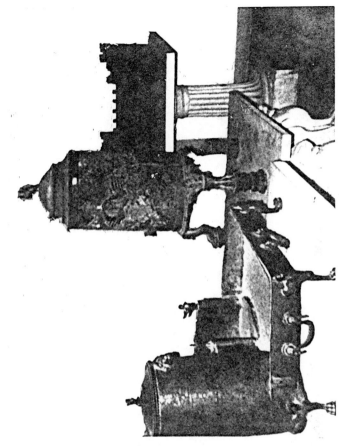

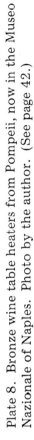

Plate 8. Bronze wine table heaters from Pompeii, now in the Museo Nazionale of Naples. Photo by the author. (See page 42.)

Plate 7. Ceramic amphora storing wine. (See page 36.)

Used with permission from Friedrich von Bassermann-Jordan; *Geschichte des Weinbaus*, Frankfurt, Anstalt, 1923, vol. 1, p. 89.

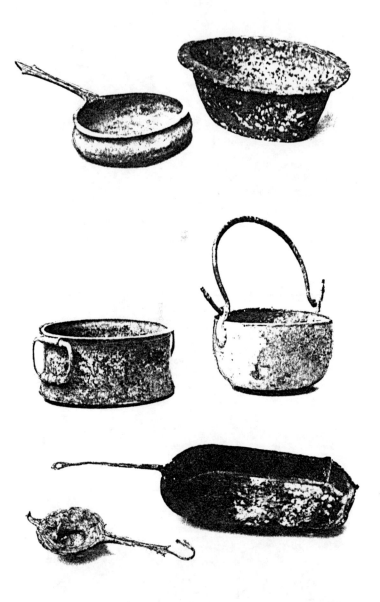

Plate 9. Roman bronze cooking pots. (See page 12.)
Courtesy of the British Museum from the Towneley Collection.

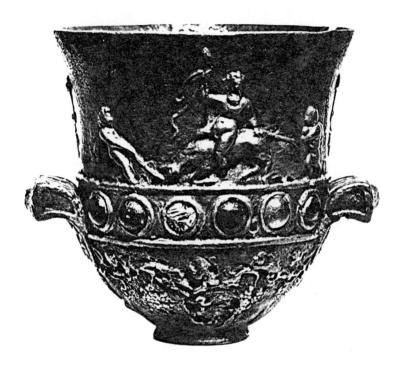

Plate 10. Lead decorative drinking cup. (See page 60.)
Courtesy of the British Museum

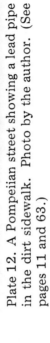

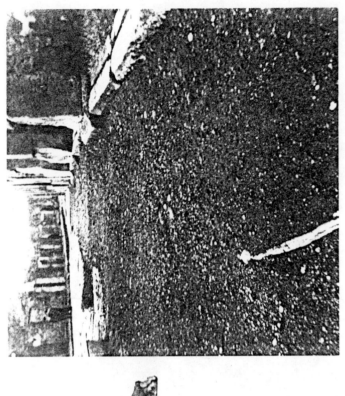

Plate 12. A Pompeiian street showing a lead pipe in the dirt sidewalk. Photo by the author. (See pages 11 and 63.)

74

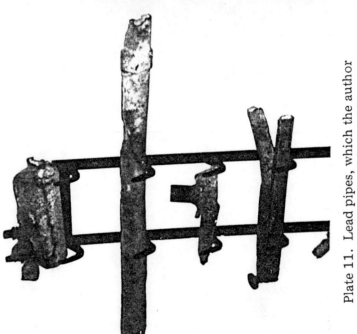

Plate 11. Lead pipes, which the author photographed in the Palermo Museum. (See pages 11 and 63.)

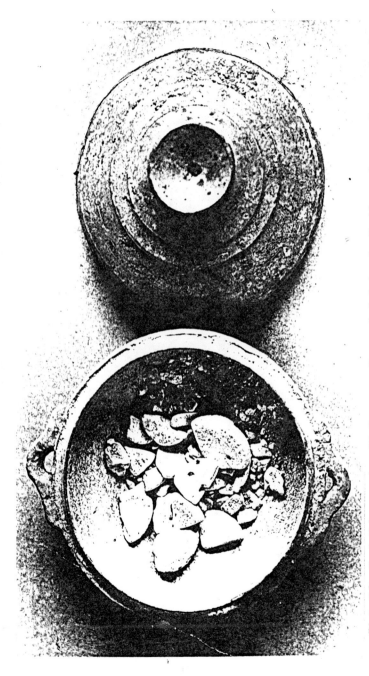

Plate 13. Corinthian *pyxis*, with its cover, from a lady's tomb. Inside are lumps of ceruse, lead carbonate face powder. (See pages 54 and 100.)

Used with permission from T. Leslie Shear: Psimythion; in *Classical Studies Presented to E. Capps*; Princeton, 1936, pages 314-317.

75

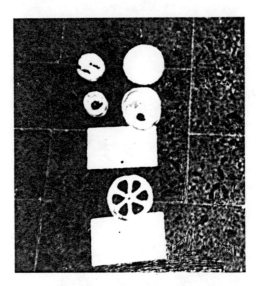

Plate 14. Lead toys, including a lead wheel, photographed by the author in the Reggio-Calabria Museum. (See page 57.)

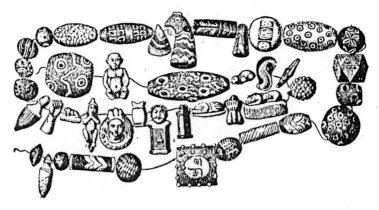

Plate 15. *Crepundia*, a child's leaden necklace. (See page 57.)
From Harold W. Johnston, *Private Life of the Romans*, 1903, page 69.

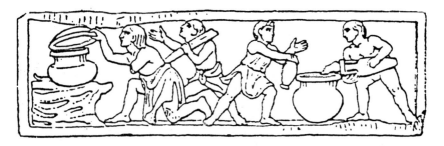

Plate 16.   An ancient relief showing must (grape juice) being boiled to make grape syrup. (See page 43.)

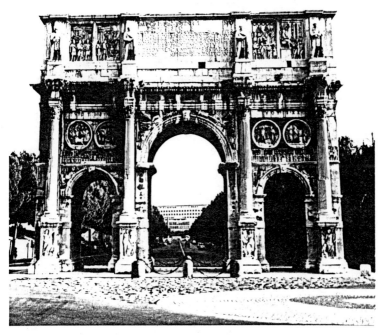

Plate 17.   The Arch of Constantine in Rome (See page 164.)

Courtesy of Al Greene & Assoc., Los Angeles.

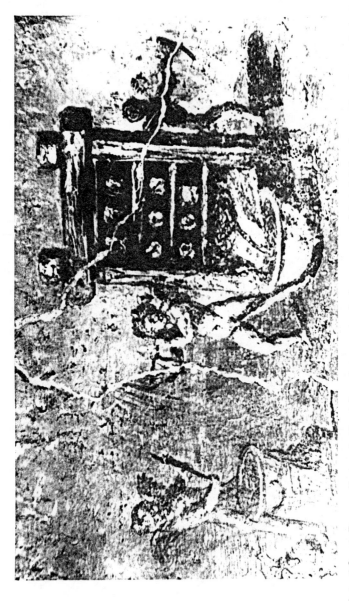

Plate 18. A Pompeiian painting showing grapes being squeezed by driving in wedges in a wine press, while on the left the must (grape juice) is being boiled and stirred. (See pages 35, 38, 43 and 165.)

Courtesy of the Superintendent of Antiquities of Campania, Museo Nazionale of Naples.

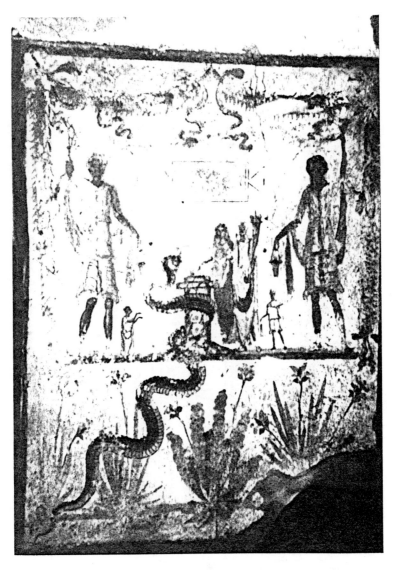

Plate 19. Wall painting in Pompeii, using much red paint.
Photo by the author. (See pages 52 and 165.)

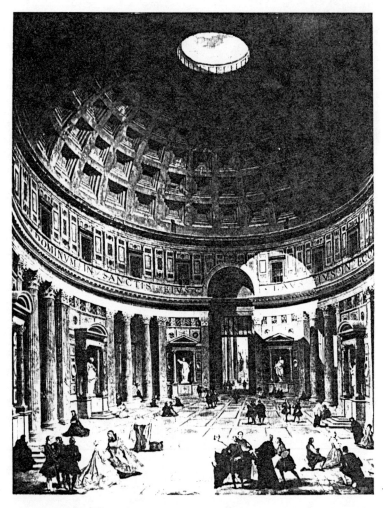

Plate 20. The Pantheon in Rome, from a painting by Giovanni
Paolo Panini, 1691-1765. (See page 164.)
Courtesy of the National Gallery of Art in Washington, D.C.

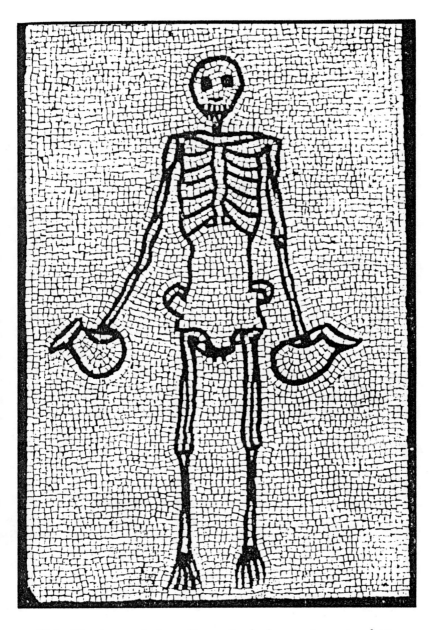

Plate 21. A mosaic from Pompeii of a banquet specter, *larva convivialis*, holding pitchers of wine. (See page 58).

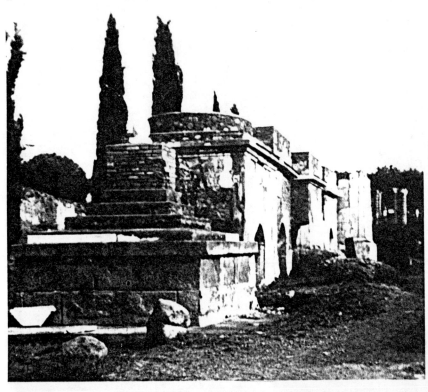

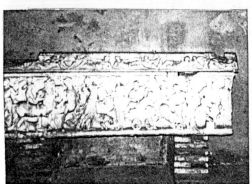

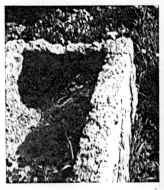

Plate 22. At top, a tomb outside Pompeii; at left, a marble coffin from Rome; and at right; a stone coffin from Agrigento, Sicily. From all these the author received bones for analysis. Photos by the author.

7

The Nature of Lead Poisoning

The purpose of this chapter is to set down the most important causes, nature, symptoms and effects of lead poisoning, as known to modern science. Our third chapter has explained how the ancients viewed and treated the malady—and so often failed to recognize or to guard aginst it. Lead's most interesting and significant aspects, for the readers of this book, are the effects it must have had on the ancients' health, sanity, and fertility, and about the ancient failure to connect these with the metal of Saturn. Today, in contrast, lead poisoning is so well known that whole books have been written about it, and governments pass laws to protect its workers and the public from it. In a single recent year, the index of the world's current medical press listed 368 articles dealing with lead poisoning.

One frustrating aspect in the diagnosis of lead poisoning, a task difficult even today, is the protean forms of this disease. A treatise on them by Aub[1] et al lists 37 symptoms, of which only two are always present in adults; and one of these is of only modern discovery—a faint blue line in the gums next to the teeth. This diversity of symptoms shows why the diagnosis was missed so often in the past, and still is sometimes. The symptoms, however conspicuous, might be of so many other diseases. Still we may say that acute plumbism in an adult is apt to present painful colic (pain in the colon or lower abdomen), constipation, and in more advanced cases local muscle paralysis, oftenest seen in a drop of the wrist, and in arthralgias (pain in the joints), or encephalopathy (convulsions or insanity). Most significant for us are its ruinous effects on fertility and sanity.

Colic and Constipation

The French physician, L. Tanquerel des Planches,* writing in 1839, was the first to devote a whole book to the history, symptoms, prognosis and treatment of acute lead poisoning. He recognized that by far the commonest presentation was with obstinate constipation and severe colic. This last acute abdominal pain was the most conspicuous symptom, seemingly centered around the navel or lower abdomen or colon, and consisting of a "violent, twisting sensation . . . (or) an acute feeling of dilaceration, tearing out, pricking, burning, boring . . ." In a severe case "the patient is a victim to the greatest anquish; the whole countenance is disturbed, the eyes hollow, dull and wandering, and the unfortunate sufferer utters the most rending cries."[2] He might press on his navel to reduce the pain, a sign that among others was recorded by the ancient medical writers. This colic is usually preceded by some days of constipation, and is frequently associated with headache and generalized muscle pains. Constipation and occasional vomiting persist thruout the duration of the colic, and vary with its intensity.[3] As serious as the colic may appear to physician and patient, the prognosis today is very good when the cause is understood, for by simply stopping further leading, and administering a chelating ("clawing") agent, usually Edathamil (EDTA), the lead atoms will be seized and withdrawn from the body. But in ancient times people not only lacked this medicine, but usually had no correct idea of the cause, unless the patient was a lead worker or had swallowed a known dose of lead or a salt of it. Table 1 on the next page shows that colic and constipation were the commonest symptoms among potters in 1910 who worked with lead glaze that would dry and be breathed or swallowed.

Anemia

Anemia is also one of the invariable accompaniments of

TABLE 1
INCIDENCE OF SYMPTOMS IN LEAD POISONING†

Symptoms	Incidence (% of cases)
Colic	73.7
Paralysis	43.5
Convulsions (encephalopathy)	24.9
Blindness, total	4.0
Blindness, partial	6.8

†From 640 cases of plumbism in Staffordshire potteries in 1910, from the data of W. D. Prendergast, reprinted in *Lead:Airborne,* * p. 153, but averaging the percent for the two sexes, which were not too different.

lead poisoning. Its victims appear pale. Pallor is not specific to plumbism, but numerous observers have described a peculiar quality of the skin that differs from that in ordinary anemia. It is variously described as "waxy, sallow complexion,"[3] or "pale or ashy-gray, with a shiny or a leaden hue, and occasionally jaundiced, yellowish tint,"[4] or "lead-colored . . . (as) transparent drapery." So Pliny* said (14:28), "From wine too comes that pallid hue, those drooping eyelids, sore eyes, tremulous hands, and insomnia." All these are symptoms of lead poisoning. So the French physician A. L. A. Fée a century and a quarter ago, with no suspicion of lead, said the ancient wines must have been somehow different from ours, since our wines make faces *red.*

Kidney Disease

In cases of long-term chronic lead poisoning, pathologists find the slow development of a contracted kidney.[5] This may progress to permanent renal disease and eventual renal failure. And it can have a result formerly much attended to: saturnine gout. Because of the renal insufficiency, uric acid cannot be excreted from the body as rapidly as formed, so it builds up. Since gout of whatever etiology is caused by uric acid buildup, it is only a matter of time before the crystals deposit in joint spaces and produce the symptoms of classic gouty disease.[6]

Blindness

Tanquerel des Planches* also mentioned that lead could result in amaurosis,[7] blindness due to causes in the central nervous system, not in the eye. His contribution to the literature can be predated by a Roman physician, who as we related in our third chapter, advised a patient who had lost the sight of one eye to stop drinking. But instead the man returned to his favorite potion. And so, "while Phryx drank wine, his eye drank poison." The ophthalmologist Rutherford[8] said that the only ingredients in spirits and wine capable of causing such optic neuritis are methyl alcohol (invented only in modern times) and lead, since "in lead poisoning there is a substantial danger of optic neuritis and atrophy."

Female Infertility

Among the many other effects of lead poisoning, acute and chronic, should be cited its many interferences with the female reproductive cycle. It causes frequent disturbances in menstruation, irregularity of the menses, amenorrhea, dysmenorrhea and menorrhagia (excessive flow).[9] The effects that most concern us are interferences with the fertility of women whom excessive lead brings to sterility, miscarriage, stillbirth, or premature labor; and children born to them are apt to die soon.

Our best evidence for the disastrous effects of lead on fertility comes not from modern medical practice, but from European medical studies of a century or more ago. By that time the disease was well understood, yet little guarded against. Many women (and men) workers in potteries, print shops and other lead trades, even if they knew they were being poisoned, kept on working from economic necessity, until they dropped in convulsions. Their condition was similar to that of the wealthier Romans, who kept on eating lead daily because they did not know what they were eating.

We cite therefore the findings of Constantin Paul,[10]

who in France in 1860 first incisively studied this subject. Among 89 lead-working women, 31 became pregnant; their 141 pregnancies led to 82 miscarriages, 4 premature births, 5 stillbirths, and 35 children who died in their first three years. Fourteen children were still living at the time of Paul's study, ten of whom were under three years of age. In all, the 141 pregnancies of 89 women would produce less than ten heirs, some of them damaged. And Paul did not count the doubtless numerous cases where lead had prevented pregnancy.

Black Teeth

The symptoms of lead poisoning are so frequently found with other conditions that lead is rarely recognized as the cause. Burton's blue line on the gums, tho never failing in adults, was, as we said at the beginning of this chapter, unknown until 1834. Black teeth are another symptom which the ancients failed to associate with lead. Their poet Horace described two young women, with black and white teeth respectively; he much preferred the one with white teeth. Black teeth should thus be a ready means for diagnosing an ancient skeleton as plumbiferous.

Lead Encephalopathy

Lead encephalopathy (convulsions or insanity) is the least common but most feared expression of acute lead poisoning. Rare among modern adults (tho it was frequent among lead-guzzling rich Romans), it hardly ever shows today in the absence of colic or paralysis. There are usually preceding complaints of headache or insomnia, effects that Athenaeus* (1:31) ascribed to certain Greek wines; or there are nightmares, depression, or ringing in the ears. Infrequently it may arise precipitously with the onset of intractable seizures, coma, or delirium.[11] Death may ensue. Today lead encephalopathy is said to occur only after prolonged, excessive exposure to airborne lead,[12] or from moonshine whiskey or most commonly in slum children eating flecks of (lead) paint from old tenement walls. Drastic poisoning may also come from habitual use of improperly fired lead-glazed ware, like some from Mexico, China or American amateur potters. Three generations ago there used to be a saying "Crazy as a painter." But today painters are more careful, and lead paints are rarely used, save on iron for its superior protection against rust.

Lead Encephalopathy in Children

Lead encephalopathy is more frequent and dangerous today among children than adults. A trait of lead poisoning constantly observed today among slum children, and probably occurring sometimes with the ancient upper class, is the impulsive mouthing or eating strange objects (pica), including paint from old tenement walls, by children of 15 to 30 months of age. The like may well have occurred too among the princelings of Rome, whose walls were lead painted, whether with works of art or plain paint, but hardly with whitewash.

Today's slum children who had been eating this lead paint from old walls become irritable, hyperactive and unable to concentrate; they tend toward violence; and perhaps they die; or what is worse, suffer permanent mental damage. This occurs to at least a quarter of those who survive acute lead encephalopathy in early childhood,[13] and to all who remain in such an environment, as would have been the ancient case. The usual sequence seems to include profound mental retardation, inability to answer questions, lack of motor coordination, and numerous other defects.[14] However, the authors Byers and Lord, have not shown that these children were average in their general nature before leading, nor in their social, racial, and genetic backgrounds. Their average I.Q. was 90.

A 1926 medical report[15] said "Of 20 child patients with lead encephalitis and convulsions . . . 13 died, 2 were left hopeless idiots, 3 are mentally retarded, 1 is mentally normal but showing ataxia, and only 1 made a complete recovery."

Among children the diagnosis of plumbism is particularly difficult, and often overlooked even today. Yet lead affects them more severely, especially by encephalopathy.[16]

For one reason, children are nearer to the ground, where kicked-up or blown heavy dust is. And babies crawl on floors, then put their dirty hands in their mouths. A study by Darrow and Schroeder[17] found the air of a minor city to contain 10.4 mg of lead per cubic meter of air at one foot elevation, 14.3 at two feet, 8.3 at five feet and 2.8 at eight feet. While the Romans had no lead from gasoline, their rich had it from many other sources, especially ceruse face powder and rouge worn by mothers and breathed by children.

The ancient ladies' ceruse face powder might well affect their infants much worse than themselves; for in the modern world this happened in Japan around 1925 and earlier, even tho such use had been discouraged since 1901. Suzuki and Kaneko[18] found lead poisoning a leading cause of death among Japanese then in Manchuria, and the fourth highest cause of infant mortality. So it was in China too. Japanese face powder and lead nipple shields were written about by Kato[19] in 1932 and Kasahara[20] in 1953. Nails darkened by lead were found even at birth. A lead ointment on the mother's breast might substitute for the lead nipple shield, to cure sores, and would be another poison to the nursling. I do not know whether the lead nipple shield was used in Roman times. Research might discover it, and if used, it would have been very poisonous.[21]

Climate is another factor. Lead poisoning in children is much more frequent in summer, due to the presence of vitamin D from sunshine, which is strong in Mediterranean lands. Vitamin D enhances the absorption of calcium, and with this might go its related element, lead.[22]

A notable consequence of acute lead poisoning in children, especially from 15 to 30 months of age, is severe brain damage.[23] Less destructive socially is a mortality rate that may reach 40 to 50 percent. Certainly in Roman times, with no understanding of causes, children remained in the deadly environment of rich homes, near the floor, and suffered the consequences to the end of their lives, long or short.

Brain Atrophy

The symptoms of plumbism, such as violence, crime,

and short attention span, would seem to spell a weakening of the person's character, will, and self-control. These virtues are functions of the *frontal and lateral lobes* of the brain, where all our life's purposes are brot together and worked out in suitable actions. It would seem worthwhile therefore to assay the frontal and the other lobes of the brains of deceased individuals who had been violent or erratic, to see if those lobes were not especially poisoned by lead. So the study of lead encephalopathy by Okazaki et al[24] found highest lead in the frontal and the hippokampal (lateral) cortices, while another study by Hamilton et al[25] on healthy brains, found the frontal lobe about average in leading. Also might be cited the work of Kato.[26] A study by Niklowitz[27] found a bulging of the soft parts of the frontal lobe of leaded infants.

In a series of papers Dr. Niklowitz analyzed the effects of massive injections of tetraethyl lead (TEL, which we have all been getting some of), on the brains of rabbits. His procedure was to give a single injection of TEL to male rabbits. After major convulsions, the animals were sacrificed, and brain tissue from the hippocampi and frontal and cerebellar cortices was subjected to electron microscopic analysis. It was found that the TEL injections induced the formation of neurofibrillary tangles of enormous length, in numerous pyramidal cells of the hippocampus and frontal cortex. Degeneration of brain cells and attack on the cell membranes are salient features of lead encephalopathia, according to these experimental results. A significant shift in the heavy metals balance within the brain also occurs—a depression in zinc level and a rise in copper level. The last may be a key element in the general insult to the brain.

Niklowitz points out that lead poisoning creates symptoms in the brain similar, if not identical, to those of Alzheimer's disease, a form of premature mental senility. But we do not seem to be dealing merely with mental deterioration and *grand mal* seizures. For example: the son of a painting contractor, who had chewed lead paint and suffered convulsions, had to be hospitalized at the age of three. Irritability and tantrums, combined with mental defect, brot about his institutionalization at age 26. An autopsy after his death 19 years later revealed that the brain was shrunken, there was a marked loss of neurones and neural sheathing, and neurofibrillary tangles were massively present. The diffuse brain atrophy found was most conspicuous in the temporal (lateral) lobes.

On the basis of his analysis of the destruction of higher control levels of the brain by lead poisoning, Dr. Niklowitz calls plumbism "the silent epidemic." Other work now in progress is searching for a link between the rising epidemic of crimes of irrational violence, and lead poisoning. Niklowitz believes that the basic processes of brain damage and destruction caused by TEL injections into rabbits, can be applied to the massive lead poisoning which especially the Roman intellectual and political elite suffered. If so, this would provide a clue to several phenomena. One would be the apparent madness of emperors such as Caligula, Nero, Commodus, and Elagabalus, some of whom seemed in their youth to be admirably fitted to rule. Another would be the sadism of the Romans, with their addiction to spectacles in which, for example, men and women were on occasion offered to famished wild beasts. A third piece of evidence would be the apparent disastrous decline of Roman intellect, mainly in the second and third centuries A.D.

Genetic Poison

Lead as a possible gene poison has been claimed by many. They argue that lead can alter the genes, the packets of heredity, and thus perhaps permanently alter future descendants, naturally changing them for the worse. Koinuma[28] found that husbands exposed to lead in a storage battery factory had 24.7 percent sterile marriages versus 14.8 percent for non-lead-workers. Stillbirths were 8.2 percent versus 2.7 percent, and infant mortality 24 percent versus 19. But in most lead trades and likely this one too, the father can bring home lead on his clothes that will reach his fmaily; and so can a breeze from a lead works. Likewise in ancient times the wife would share the husband's drinks and foods, and he could absorb some of her cosmetics.

Arthralgia

Tanquerel des Planches* observed that lead's arthralgic pain attacked any of the joints, but more frequently those in the lower limbs. He described it as a sharp, burning, boring, or simply numbing pain, that could radiate out and encompass the overlying tissue. He made an important differential diagnostic point when he explained that unlike rheumatoid arthritis (with which this might be mistaken) lead arthralgia causes no swelling nor redness. In addition, the leaded patient is constantly moving around, trying to find a comfortable position, something never seen in arthritics, who prefer to remain still.

Another of the most characteristic signs among lead workers today is the "wrist drop," a motor paralysis observed among lead workers. But it is hardly ever seen in children.

Atmospheric Lead

H. D. Bryce-Smith tells of lead pollution from petrol,[29] both from leaded gasoline burnt to the oxide, and from the worse, organo-lead compounds that might be obtained from the unburned leaded gasoline around garages, or sometimes sniffed as a vice. Atmospheric lead in our cities some years ago was increasing at five percent a year, a fact that certainly demanded the deleading of gasoline, which is now nearly accomplished. There was no organo-lead in Roman times. With Waldron, the same author[30] shows connections of lead poisoning with violence, hooliganism, and crime. Symptoms include excitement, insomnia, hallucinations, impaired memory, loss of concentration and short attention span. Those authors conclude that probably more than a quarter of the children affected will be left with permanent damage.

Animal Experimentation

Perhaps the best evidence on lead poisoning must come from animals, who can be freely experimented on, and protected from all *environmental* leading of their offspring.

Such evidence has been gathered by numerous scientists named in *Lead, Airborne** (pp. 166. 169), and accredited by Harriet L. Hardy,[31] an authority on the subject. Stöfen[32] also tells of bulls pastured on lead-dusted grass losing their fertility. Numerous experiments with small male animals leaded in a laboratory showed sharply reduced fertility, and in some cases *alterations in their spermatozoa.*[33] Teratogenic effects, producing offspring of abnormal form, indicating alterations of the genes, have been proved by experiments on three species of rodents.[34] Such effects from lead would not have been so harmful in Roman times as today, because the ancients more than we allowed infanticide for the misbegotten, a race-purifying institution. Schwantiz et al[35] have written of damage to the chromosomes, affecting their splitting, among lead workers. Reduced libido and sexual potency are other lead effects claimed.

The Metabolism of Lead

There are two major portals thru which lead is introduced into the body; the mouth and the nose. Ingestion and inhalation are of very different significance, because it has been determined that only about 10 percent of ingested lead is absorbed by the intestines, while 25-50 percent or more of inspired lead is absorbed by the body. In addition, the lead that is not immediately breathed out may be wafted upward by the cilia all the way to the throat, where it can be swallowed and then processed like lead eaten. Most of the lead abosrbed under normal conditions was eaten, simply because we eat much more of it than we breathe and retain. Studies of the average diet of Americans show that we daily ingest approximately 0.33 mg. of lead in our food, especially from leafy vegetables and sea food, since in recent centuries the air and the upper layers of the ocean have become polluted by man-produced lead. While we Americans are daily ingesting a third of a milligram in our food, we are breathing in

---

34. But as to whether the leading of an animal can produce a permanent, racial change in its descendants, we have not found conclusive evidence. The elaborate experiments of Colin on guinea-pigs seemed to deny this.

and retaining only .03 mg. Applying the above absorption
intakes it follows that roughly forty micrograms (0.04 mg.)
are actually absorbed daily. The rest is promptly excreted,
thru the bile and feces chiefly, but some thru the urine and a
very little thru sweat and hair. There remains only enough
net absorption in the average "non-poisoned" person to give
blood lead levels of about 15-40 micrograms per 100 ml. of
blood. Dr. Kehoe in his monumental studies on lead metabolism, concluded that most of the ingested lead (approximately 0.33 mg/day) is excreted directly in the feces without ever
having been absorbed. While there is no proof that lead at
such blood levels, 15-40 micrograms per 100 ml. of blood, is
dangerous, acutely or chronically, it is probably all a little
harmful, since no one has ever proved any *good* in lead. As
Patterson* shows from his glacial measurements, we are all
getting far more of it environmentally than the percentage
found in the surface of the earth, and far more than two or
three thousand years ago, since airborne lead has greatly increased in the last two centuries.

In an experiment extended over five years, Kehoe studied the effect on several people of ingesting approximately
1.3 mg. of lead per day. He analyzed the excreta (feces and
urine) during that whole time and finally concluded that the
total positive lead added to the body was a mere 110 mg. At
no time were there signs or symptoms of lead poisoning, and
no adverse effects on the subjects were observed.[36] But Dr.
Kehoe was forced to concede that amounts ingested at that
level could very well have resulted in lead poisoning if there
had occurred an important precipitating event, such as an
acidic condition that mobilized lead from the bones, or an increased acute ingestion.[37] This observation meets with con-
currence by Chisolm, who has stated "Lead intoxication results from *chronic* increased ingestion of lead . . . repetitive
ingestion or inhalation of small amounts of lead is usually
far more dangerous than a single massive exposure.[38]

While there is today some controversy about the relative
importance of breathed compared to ingested lead, Kehoe's
studies indicate that most of what is absorved has been eaten.
Patterson* in particular pointed to the danger from inspired

lead thru additives in gasoline, sometimes in their deadlier liquid, organo-lead form, and said they may be crucial for people living in dense urban areas or near an auto highway. But such gasoline is now mostly banned.

Tho there was no tetraethyl lead in Roman times, there was lead breathed from cosmetics, burnt wood, and sometimes from hot lead. We cited the study by Darrow and Schroeder[39] concerning the air quality of the main street of Brattleboro, Vermont. This study found two or three times as much lead at the level of a child as at an adult's level. Lead from Roman paints, dust, and especially cosmetics must have likewise reached the children who are particularly susceptible.

Another portal of entry for lead may be the skin. Some medical literature on this matter offers experimental evidence that lead is not absorbed thru the skin, even if rubbed in, while other clinical data indicate this as the only possible entry. But all researchers will allow that lead can be absorbed thru ulcers, sores, or other openings of the skin. In ancient times lead salts were recommended by physicians for healing such ulcers or wounds. And indeed they were effective against the infection, because of their sterilizing effect. But they also entered the bloodstream. The ancients furthermore used much lead in contraceptive vaginal douches, and eye washes, which were partly taken into the body. It has been suggested that inorganic lead salts, if suspended in a lipid (fat, greasy) medium for lead, must be applied over a very long time to be of any consequence. But the lead face powder, ceruse, can be easily *breathed* in, and reach an infant. And minium (lead) rouge, or lead *kohl* for darkness about the eyes, may well enter mouth or eyes. There have been a number of clinical accounts of acute lead poisoning, in which the only exposure to lead was that of cosmetics, or toilet articles like the leaden containers the ancient ladies used.[40] Another article[41] tells of the deaths of four women in one modern family from using a lead-carbonate-based face powder ("Flaky White"), the ancients' ceruse, while their husbands and relatives who lived with them showed no signs of lead intoxication.

If lead is indeed absorbed thru the skin, its method of

ingress is unknown.

But well known are the methods of inspiration and ingestion. When lead enters the lungs and is implanted on the walls of the alveoli, cells move out from the tissue and phagocytize (ingest) the lead. It is then transferred directly to the general circulation, thus avoiding passage thru the purifying liver. All nutrients absorbed thru the gastrointestinal tract drain via the portal system to the liver, where the lead is taken up and largely excreted in the bile.[42] Hence lead breathed is far more harmful, gram for gram, than the same amount eaten.

Lead eaten or drunk follows closely the physiology of calcium absorption. In fact, because of competition between these two elements, it has been noted that lead taken with large amounts of calcium will not be so well absorbed, but more fully excreted. As with calcium metabolism, an increased level of vitamin D, which enhances the absorption of calcium, also heightens that of lead.[43] Hence comes its far greater severity for children enjoying summer sunshine.

Once absorbed into the bloodstream, the lead is transported, like calcium, by complexing with the blood albumin or with the red blood cells. From the blood, lead may be excreted in the urine, sweat, or bile, or deposited in the bone as a lead fosfate. However, the chemical properties must be very precise for bone deposition; the blood pH must be between 7.4 and 7.8.[44] A pH of 7.4 is normal for the blood, so under normal conditions lead goes into the bones. If the blood pH falls below 7.4, a condition known as acidosis is present, and under these circumstances the lead may be mobilized from the bone and back into the bloodstream. Lead here may upset the delicate balance the body tries to preserve, and bring on the pathologic symptoms of acute plumbism. Such a condition as acidosis can occur under many different disease states (especially infections), after prolonged, severe exercise or work, or by alcoholism.[45] So if a person chronically exposed to increased amounts of lead goes on an alcoholic binge, as the Roman wealthy men often did, an acute attack of lead poisoning becomes likely.[45]

There are two major means by which lead interferes

with normal biochemical pathways. It seems to replace one-for-one the copper in brain nervous tissue. This copper is usually complexed with enzymes found at the nerve terminal or in the mitochondria of the cell. In fact, detailed studies of the lead-poisoned cell have exhibited cytopathologic changes and lesions, preferential to the nerve cell mitochondria.[46] These findings have prompted one investigator to conclude: "The specific property of lead, therefore, in regard to its toxic mechanism, is its ability to interfere competitively with the metal components of metal ligands of the nerve cells."[47] How this actually develops into the symptoms of plumbism is not known.

The second major effect biochemically is the inhibition of some of the steps in the manufacture of the central component of hemoglobin, the heme molecule.[48] This is the first morphologic sign of any injury due to lead. How lead actually damages the red cell is not known—it may be due to changes in heme production or it may be due to interference with calcium at the cell wall. In any case, the red cell life span is shortened and bone marrow production of new cells simply cannot maintain a normal complement of cells. This is why, invariably, lead-poisoned people are found to be anemic. In addition, with biochemical tests, the urine can be examined for one of the products of heme synthesis—delta amino-levulinate. Indeed, this biosynthetic pathway is so sensitive to the toxic effects of lead that two of the metabolites, delta aminolevulinate and coproporphyrin, can be consistently demonstrated in great excess in the urine, even in the absence of clinical symptoms.[49] The interference with heme production has other effects as well, since the erythrocyte is not the only cell with a heme pathway. All cells synthesize their own heme enzymes (including catalase, and cytochromes that are involved in energy production in the cell), and this may be another system in which inhibition by lead could disrupt the cell membrane.[50]

The pathologists of plumbism always recall that if the patient refrains from further contact with lead he will soon get better. This is obviously because his excretion of lead can then overtake his past absorption. Excretion of earlier absorbed lead occurs chiefly via the feces, just as happens to most of the lead when originally eaten.[51] The portion of it absorbed by the intestine goes to the liver in the portal system, and is mostly taken up and re-excreted into the intestinal tract in the bile. The urine serves to cleanse the blood, so that as the blood level of lead goes up, the amounts excreted in the urine do also.[52] But they are always much less than that excreted in the feces. These processes apparently have the capacity to increase their role, because there is some suggestion that as long periods of time pass, with constant exposure to high levels of lead, the excretory processes become relatively more important, in an attempt to balance the intake.[53] In addition, there is some lead excreted in the sweat, probably as much as in the urine.

These then are our major means for getting rid of lead under normal conditions. However, it is also proved that during lactation, lead is excreted in human breast milk.[54] This is of great pertinence to us because it represents a direct means of passing lead to a child at his most susceptible age.

Finally, this section on the metabolism of lead must deal with the action of acute as compared to chronic intoxication by lead. We have mentioned the studies by Kehoe suggesting that the average American intake is 0.33 mg of lead per day, that ingestion of 0.6 mg/day would not constitute a significant insult, and that ingestion of 1.3 mg/day for five years results in a relatively mild lead buildup (which may only have significance under certain circumstances). It is then apparent that the chronic ingestion of somewhat modest amounts of lead in the adult is not associated with any distinct symptoms of plumbism. The importance of the insult, however, seems to go up exponentially once it climbs much above that level of 1.3 mg/day. For instance, it has been demonstrated that a daily intake of 2.5 mg required some four years for toxic effects, while a daily intake of 3.5 mg required only a few months.[54] Presumably this is because the lead simply cannot be excreted, nor deposited in the bones, fast enough to prevent the poisonous effects. This has been noted from the amount of lead present in skeletal bone as related to the length of lead exposure. "When the lead content of the skeleton is found to be high and that in the soft tissues relatively low, the time involved in the absorptive process was relatively long.[55] The opposite occurs in cases of acute poisoning, especially as found in children.

Lead Poisoning in Modern Industry

Lead poisoning is still important today, probably our number one industrial disease, altho strongly combatted there. About 170 articles a year on it are indexed from the world's medical press. It has become rarely fatal in industry, because of constant vigilance there, even if not among slum children. Today workers are not only watched out for, but when found leaded are promptly yanked off the job, and the lead extracted from them by a chelating (grasping) chemical, usually EDTA (Edathamil). Even by Tanquerel des Planches'* time only 2.3 percent of those recognized as so afflicted died.[56]

The Historians of Lead Poisoning

The only full history of this major disease which we have found, has unfortunately not yet been published, tho photocopies from it can be bought. Lloyd G. Stevenson,* M.D., PhD.: *A History of Lead Poisoning.* Like us he has made abundant use of the discoveries of Hofmann* and Kobert* as to ancient times. These physicians were on the edge of our discovery, yet did not fully grasp it, when they mentioned the empty cradles of the Roman aristocracy, as proof of the devastation from ancient lead.

A brief treatment of ancient plumbism we have mentioned from Tanquerel des Planches.* Louis Levin: *die Gifte in der Weltgeschichte*, 1920, 596 pages, covers little save malicious poisoning.

Lead poisoning in the ancient world has been recently treated by Waldron,[57] and the story of the recognition of lead's relation to fertility in the 19th century was first well treated by Denuefbourg[58] in 1905. And an historical article was written by the physician McCord in 1953,[59] adding further medical explanation.

1. J. C. Aub, L. T. Fairhall, A. S. Minot & P. Reznikoff: *Lead Poisoning*, 265 pp., 1926.
2. Tanquerel des Planches,* pp. 73-4.
3. *Lead, Airborne,** p. 85.
4. Cantarow & Trumper,* p. 59.
5. Ibid, p. 94.
6. *Lead, Airborne,** pp. 114-5.
7. Tanquerel des Planches,* p. 202.
8. W. J. Rutherford: Lead Poisoning in the First Century: *British Jol. of Ophthal.*, 18:36-8, 1934, citing Martial: *Epigrams*, VI:78.
9. Cantarow & Trumper,* p. 84.
10. Paul, Constantin: Etude sur l'intoxication lente par les preparations de plomb . . . sur le produit de la conception: *Archives gén. de méd.*, 1860, pp. 513-33.
11. *Lead, Airborne,** p. 87.
12. Ibid, p. 88.
13. J. J. Chisolm & Eugene Kaplan: Lead Poisoning in Childhood; comprehensive mgmt. and prevention: *Jol. Pediat.*, 73:942-50 (1968), p. 946; and *Lead, Airborne,** p. 95.
14. *Lead, Airborne,** pp. 95-8.
15. H. B. Wilcox & J. P. Caffey Lead Poisoning in Nursing Infants, *Jol. Amer. Med. Asn.*, 86:1514-6, p. 1514.
16. Jane S. Lin-Fu: Undue Absorption of Lead among Children, a new look at an old problem: *New Engl. Jol. of Med.*, 286:702-9.
17. D. K. Darrow and H. A. Schroeder: Childhood Exposure to Environmental Lead, Abstracts of papers, Amer. Chem. Soc., 166th meeting, 1973, p. AGFD 060.
18. T. Suzuki & J. Kaneko: Serous Meningitis in Infants Caused by Lead Poisoning from White Powders: *Jol. of Oriental Med.*, 9:55-66, 1925.
19. K. Kato: Lead Meningitis in Infants: *Amer. Jol. of Diseases of Children*, 44:569-91, 1932, p. 580.
20. M. Kasahara: *Lead Poisoning in Sucklings*, 1953, about p.35. He also cites L. E. Holt & McIntosh: *Holt's Diseases of Infancy and Childhood*, 10th ed., 1936.
21. Wilcox & Caffey, supra.
22. *Lead, Airborne,** p. 167.
23. Chisolm & Kaplan, supra, p. 956.
24. H. Okazaki & Aronson, DiNatale & Olvera: Acute Lead Encephalopathy: *Trans. of Amer. Neurolog. Asn.*, 88:248-50, 1963.
25. E. I. Hamilton, M. J. Minski & J. J. Cleary: The Concentration and Distribution of Some Stable Elements in Healthy Human Tissues: *Science of the Total Environment*, I:341-74, 1973.

26. Kato, supra.
27. W. J. Niklowitz: Lead, a Cause of Neurofibrillary Changes: *Jol. of Neuropathology and Exper. Neurol.*, Jan. 1976, p. 103, etc.
28. S. Koinuma: Japan Letter, *Jol. Amer. Med. Asn.*, 86; p. 1924 in 1926, quoted by Alice Hamilton & Harriet L. Hardy; *Indus. Toxicology*, 2nd ed., 1949.
29. D. Bryce-Smith: Lead Pollution from Petrol: *Chemistry in Britain*, 7:284-6, 1971.
30. D. Bryce-Smith & H. A. Waldron: Lead, Behaviour and Criminality: *Ecologist*, 4:367-77, 1974.
31. U. S. Public Health Service: *Symposium on Environmental Lead Contamination*. On damage to heredity see Harriet L. Hardy in pp. 73-83.
32. D. Stöfen: die Sowjetische Toxikologie, ihre Probleme: *Chem. Ztg.*, 1969, pp. 966-8, esp. 966. Cf. also his Scarcely Regarded European Papers on Lead, at the Intnatl. Symposium on Environmental Health Aspects of Lead, at Amsterdam, 1972. And his die larvierte Bleivergiftung: *Archiv für Hyg. u. Bakteriol.*, 152:5;6,68, pp. 551-8, with translated summaries.
33. E. C. Colin: Comparison of the Descendants of Lead-poisoned Male Guinea-pigs; *Jol. of Experimental Zool.*, 60:427-84, 1931. Adds human data from C. Paul (see Note 10 above).
    G. Dalldorf: Impairment of Reproduction in Rats by Ingestion of Lead: *Science*, 102:670-1, Dec. 28, 1945. First generation.
    D. Stöfen: Larvierte Bleivergiftung-ein Massenphänomen? *Selekia*, 12:37, Sept. 14, 1970, incl. dangers to the race on last page.
34. See the note on page 77.
35. G. Schwanitz & Lehnert & Gebhart: Chromosomenschaden bei beruflicher Bleibelastung: *Deutsch Med. Wochenschr.*, 95:1636 -40 (1970). Includes secondary chromosomal aberrations and English summary.
    Lead, Airborne, * p. 166, and V. H. Ferm & S. J. Carpenter: Developmental malformations resulting from administration of lead salts: *Exp. Molec. Path.*, 7:208-13, 1967.
36. Robert H. Kehoe: The Metabolism of Lead in Man in Health and Disease: *Jol. Royal Inst. Pub. Health*, 24:101-20, 1961.
37. Ibid, p. 195.
38. Chisolm & Kaplan, supra, p. 944.
39. Darrow & Schroeder, supra.
40. Wilcox & Caffey, supra.
41. Moses Barron & Harold Habein: Lead Poisoning, with Special References to Poisoning from Lead Cosmetics: *Amer. Jol. of Med. Sci.*, 162:833-61, 1921, p. 840.

42. Alice Hamilton & Harriet L. Hardy: *Indus. Toxicology*, Hoeber pub., NY, 1949, p. 62.

43. *Lead, Airborne,** p. 167.

44. Kato, supra, p. 526.

45. Ibid., p. 526. Also Hamilton & Hardy, supra, p. 65.

46. Werner J. Niklowitz & David W. Yeager: Interference of Pb with Essential Brain Tissue, Cu, Fe and Zn: *Life Sci.*, 13:897-905 (1973), p. 903.

47. Ibid, p. 902.

48. J. J. Chisolm: Disturbances in the Biosynthesis of Heme in Lead Intoxication, *Jol. Pediat.*, 64:179.

49. Ibid, p. 174.

50. Ibid, 179.

51. Ibid, p. 179.

52. Hamilton & Hardy, supra, p. 62.

53. Cantarow & Trumper,* pp. 6-7.

54. L. S. Goodman & Al. Gilman: *Pharmacological Basis of Therapeutics*, Macmillan, NY, 1970, p. 979.

55. Kehoe, supra, p. 183.

56. J. J. Chisolm: Disturbances in the Biosynthesis of Heme in Lead Intoxication, *Jol. Pediat.*, 64:179.

57. R. A. Waldron: Lead Poisoning in the Ancient World: *Medical Hist.*, 17:391-9, Oct. 1973.

58. Henri Deneufbourg: *De l'Intoxication saturnine dans ses rapports avec la grossesse*, 108 pp., 1905, a thesis at the Univ. of Paris.

59. C. P. McCord: Lead and Lead Piping in Early America: *Indus. Med. & Surgery*, serially in vols. 22 and 23, 1953, 4.

8

Their Bones:
the Proofs by Clinical
Necromancy

Let us now add the evidence of Clinical Necromancy. Necromancy is the old art of calling up the dead and questioning them—a great art for the historian *if he can work it*. And as we shall show, it has been worked on our problem by others and now by us, who have called up the dead in the form of their bones, and have questioned them by analyses of their bones for lead. But previous necromancers were not working on the class angle, to test the *dysgenic* effect of ancient lead poisoning. Nor did the earlier chemists possess the accurate modern techniques that Professor Clair C. Patterson, and separately the Kettering Laboratory, have employed for our own research.

Rudolf Kobert* summoned 22 people from the ancient world, in the form of their bones, and his student Rosenblatt* found lead in two from Roman Carthage and two from the same city before the Roman conquest, including a child in a stone coffin (hence rich), who was badly leaded. The other 18 cases came from outside the Empire, in time or place, and could show no lead, altho five early ones showed tin or copper. The chemistry of 1906 hardly permitted more

†The author has been greatly assisted in this chapter, and in Appendices A and B, by Professor Clair C. Patterson, and his laboratory at the California Institute of Technology in Pasadena, California.

accuracy in such cases than saying whether the metal was de-
tected or not. A few years later the dithizone colorimetric,
and recently the spectrographic methods, have enabled far
more sensitive and accurate analyses for lead. So in 1959 the
German necromancers W. Specht and K. Fischer[1] called up
Pope Clement II, who had died in Rome in 1047, after only a
ten-month reign, and was buried in a stone coffin. They
found so much lead, 500 ppm (parts per million of dried
bone) in his one surviving bone, a rib, that he must have died
of lead poisoning. This tends to confirm old contemporary
suspicions that he was poisoned "by a person or persons unknown" because the emperor Henry II had forced him on the
college of cardinals.[2]

Another recent and striking use of lead clinical necromancy to explain history was reported in 1969 when two
Russian necromancers Prozorovsky and Kolosova[3] called up
Tsar Ivan IV, the Terrible, who died in 1584, as well as his
two sons and a concerned nobleman. They found enough
lead in Ivan to explain the crazy cruelty of his later reign. His
sons were even more heavily leaded, which could explain the
insanity of his successor Fyodor, and the prior death of Ivan's
elder son. His father who loved him had killed him on im-
pulse, by repeated blows with his iron-tipped staff, when the
son asked to lead an army. Earlier that day the Tsar had beat-
en this son's pregnant wife for a most trivial error. There
were also considerable mercury and arsenic in the elder son.

Still another use of lead clinical necromancy was by Dr.
Jarcho,[4] who found 9-17 ppm of lead in the bones of five
pre-historic thirteenth-century Indians of Arizona, who used
lead-glazed pottery, and found somewhat less in six bones
from the tribe that had made the ware.

Other cases include finds of entombed skeletons of fine
ladies of ancient Athens and Corinth, with lead in their
bones, still guarding their beauty secret, ceruse face powder,
in lumps of the lead salt in a graceful pottery *pyxis.* One of

2.   After a brief replacement by Benedict IX the Emperor forced in
      a substitute, Damasus II. But he died after only 23 days. There-
      after the Emperor seems to have run out of candidates, and the
      independence of the Cardinals was vindicated.

these is illustrated in Plate 13 on page 75.

I also have been gathering, with much travel and expense, bones from the Roman Empire after 150 B.C., and some from Greek and other lands before and after our formal epoch. I have had 134 bone analyses made for their lead content, to add to our thesis the evidence of clinical necromancy. While some bones have been obtained by correspondence, most have been acquired by personal visits to museums of archeology, especially from Italy, and from the British Museum of Science in London. My special thanks go to Don R. Brothwell of the last, to Dr. J. Lawrence Angel at the Smithsonian Institution in Washington, to the officials in Rome, Naples and Pompeii, to Prof. Melchiorre Masali of Turin, Dr. Maria Guinovart of the Archaeological Museum in Tarragona, Spain, and to Prof. Carlo Maxia of the University at Cagliari, Sardinia, as well as to many others named in the Appendices.

The Problem of the Which-Bone Factor

A scientist who has whole skeletons available can learn all sorts of facts about those people's lives, as shown in the books we have starred on this subject by Brothwell* and by Wells.*

But there are problems of clinical necromancy that have not been dealt with by any of our predecessors, problems we have labored on for years, for their probable effects and relation to our results. For our special problem—to measure the particular, distinctive dose of lead poison in different types of long-dead people, by a single bone fragment from each one, given us at random—is a problem that has never been taken up before, unless perhaps by two Russian women whose work in 1959 we have not been able to find.[5] But we have spent much time attacking these problems, which we shall explain presently as well as in our Appendices A-C, and give our best solutions.

A principal problem the author faced was the unequal proclivity of the different bones of the body to store lead. So he spent perhaps a year in searching the medical literature in all important languages in order to find articles (17 listed in Appendix C) in which more than one bone from the same body had been assayed for lead. In this way he could then judge the relative proclivity of the different bones for taking up lead. He found there cited 1,452 such bone pairs in which one of the bones was a rib. There were 168 cases in which a rib and a vertebra had been analyzed (from the same cadaver).

Taking the leading of the rib for our standard of reference, the author found a vertebra part to have on average 1.37 times as heavy a proportion of lead as the same person's rib; so we have listed a "Which-bone Factor" of the vertebra as 1.37. The same was done with 12 other bones in our Table 4 in Appendix C on page 202. This Table also tells the number of bone pairs on which each ratio was based.

However, for 7 seldom-analyzed bones, he could find no comparison with that person's rib. But he did find comparisons with other bones and these seldom-analyzed bones. That meant a comparison could be made with another bone whose rib ratio had been estimated. Thus we can get a rib ratio indirectly, by dividing the other bone's leading by the other-bone/rib ratio, so as to get its degree of leading in terms of our common denominator, namely, how much lead it would have held had it been a rib.

Admittedly our procedure is somewhat inaccurate because of our scantiness of comparisons in most cases, and because of lead's manner of deposit. For it tends to settle first in the porous bones (including ribs, vertebra, sternum, cranium, and ends of long bones), which all have a circulation of blood, and later to migrate into the dense, tubular, shaft bones, where it settles in the almost insoluble and hence harmless form of lead trifosfate, and accumulates thruout life.

The Problem of the Age Factor

We have stiriven also to cope with the age factor in the numerous cases where the age of our bone-person is known, even if but roughly. For the age of the individual makes a wide difference in the significance of his lead burden. So we have set up in Appendix B the following scheme for coping with the problem, whenever we have any indication of the person's age. This is necessary because the percentage of lead in bones tends to pile up with his age. That which would be only average in an adult's bone would be far above normal in a child, and would probably indicate he died of the plumbic poisoning.

Several scientists have provided lead-in-bone analyses of ordinary people today. Their tables show the average leading of their standard bones according to age at death (from whatever cause). We should particularly cite the data from Barry and Mossman[6] from whom we have redrawn by permission, in our Table 2 on the next page one regression line for lead in the tibias (shank bones), giving equal weight to the two sexes. These tibias can probably represent life's leading rate for all the dense, tubular bones. Our second, the curved line, drawn freehand from data in Schroeder and Tipton,[7] Krause,[8] Jaworowski,[9] Morris,[10] and Nusbaum,[11] shows an average course for lead accumulating in the *porous* bones, such as ribs.

Our Statistical Methods for Dealing with the Age Factor

If we have only indications that the person was adult, we do nothing save to record his leading with correction for the Which-bone Factor. We assume that he died when average adults did, say around 45. But if we have any better indication of age, we spot it (corrected for the Which-bone Factor), on the appropriate graph in Table 2, for dense or for porous bones. Suppose he were a child two years old and

6. P. S. E. Barry & D. B. Mossman: Lead Concentrations in Human Tissue: *British Jol. of Indus. Med.*, 27:339-51, 1970; using their Fig. 1. From post-mortems in an English industrial area. Of 43 men only 4 had known exposures to lead. The men's tibias had 30 percent more of lead than the 30 women averaged. Our one regression line was drawn midway between the two sexes; and its starting point moved a very little, to start at 0 for both age and lead.

11. R. E. Nusbaum et al, as sources for Which-bone data, their Table 5. Rib and calvarium were rather similar, peaking at age 45.

TABLE 2: LEAD IN DENSE AND POROUS BONES,
ACCORDING TO AGE*

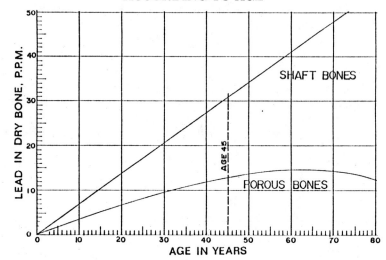

*From P. S. E. Barry and D. B. Mossman, Lead Concentrations in Hu-
an Tissues, *British Jol. of Indus. Med.*, 27:339-51, 1970, Fig. 1, com-
bining its regression lines for 39 men and 26 women, with equal weight
in each sex.

---

had 5 ppm of lead. For an adult that would be but minor
leading. But for a two-year-old it would be so noxious that it
likely killed the child; hence it should be reckoned as very
severe in calculating our averages for survival of rich and
poor. We can do this by assuming that the child continued to
live and pack lead into that bone at the drastically lethal rate
charted on one of our two standard slopes, until he/she
reached that standard age of 45 for death. So if it were a
porous bone, where lead goes in and out, we should follow a-
long the lower, curving line. This line rises 6.5-fold higher at
age 45 than at age 2; so the child's leading at our standard
age of 45 should be manyfold higher than when he or she was
2. But if the bone was a dense, tubular one, like the tibia, its
leading would have soared 15-fold, namely, to 30. (But in
any case we would have already applied the Which-bone
Factor.)

One might still ask: But why attach such importance to an event that never happened, his dying at 45? The answer, Because thus our statistics will reflect the vital, weighty fact that he died too young, while children much less leaded lived on to a normal age for their death.

Only by thus considering the age and the class of bone (lead-keeping or lead-porous) can the doubtless numerous cases of death in youth or childhood by lead poisoning be given their true significance. Without such statistical treatment our cases of people who died young—with so few ppm of lead, yet facing a ruinous load later from taking it in a fatal rate—such people would have been reckoned as cases of light leading.

Still if some scientist does not approve of our procedures he can rather easily substitute other methods of calculation, in this and many other matters, while still utilizing our bone analyses data. Our precedures are further explained in Appendices A to C.

The Problem of Averaging

One statistical problem of averaging might be called that of overkill—lead findings so large, running into hundreds or even thousands of ppm of lead, that they would have been more than enough to kill the person; yet he was only one fatality. We have dealt with this problem by the statisticians' device of using for our average not the ordinary arithmetic mean, but the *median*, which is the size of the *middle item*. (If the count of items is an even number, then we average the middle two.) The median average gives little weight to the exceptionally large items, the overkill in our own case. For each of these items will only move the median one-half step higher by its presence. Still we put the extraordinary assays in our record, for what they may be worth to some later student.

Description of Appendices A and B

So we have collected and had analyzed by the two lead-

ing laboratories of the nation for such studies, 134 bones
from 125 people, besides a few food items from ancient
times whose leading we also had measured. We present all
these findings in Appendix B.

However, first our Appendix A gives detailed explanations of how the analyses were made and presented in Appendix B, including the laboratory methods, our system, and the
abbreviations used in reporting the findings.

In Appendix B the bones and other assayed objects have
been divided into six groups, lettered A to F, the more co-
gent groups being listed first. We report for each bone usually its date, country, donor, analysis number, laboratory that
analyzed it, which bone of the body it was, how much lead
it contained in ppm (parts per million by weight) of dried
bone, and how much lead it would have held had it been a
rib.   If the person's age is known, that factor is reckoned
with.

In this Appendix B, the first and chief section is Group
A, which lists bones from within the Roman Empire in space
and time, and whose social class (rich, middle class, or poor)
is inferrable from the conditions of the burials.   Group B
next covers a few ancient bones from outside the Empire in
space or time, whose social class is known.   Group C contains
those from the Empire but not identifiable by class; Group D
comprises such from outside the Empire; Group E contains
bones analyzed but not further calculated because of some
disturbing factor, usually cremation; and Group F lists food
objects containing lead.

At the end of each group the count of people tested is
given, including cases where more than one bone was analyzed
from a body.   The lead averages for each of the three social
classes are computed for Group A only (averages per person,
not per bone).

Our Social Class Averages

Therefore, we have computed some social class averages
for the Roman Empire in space and time from Group A. We
find in our 15 rich people a median average of 80 ppm of

lead, compared with a median of 27 ppm for our seven middle class folk, and 34.5 for our 24 poor (not including the Emporion group of lead workers, or 36 if we include one median Emporion case). The lead level of the Roman poor is similar to that in industrial nations today, but the 3-fold higher level of the Roman rich is sufficient to produce life-threatening dysfunctions, including sterility and insanity, on a widespread basis among the rich.

A source of possible error in our analyses could be the movement of lead into the bones after death thru ground water circulating around burial artifacts and then into the bones. Thus the high level of lead in the Roman rich could have come partly from this source. It should be made clear that when the bones were analyzed by the California Institute of Technology, corrections were made for any lead found in the dirt attached to the bone, but not for any lead that might have been chemically added to the bone from soil moisture or water. However, there is one way to deduce whether lead had been chemically added to the bones after death—that is, by examining the *copper* levels in the bones. Since the Romans, both rich and poor, and the peoples coming before and after the Roman era, all knew about copper poisoning and generally avoided it, then all those peoples would probably have about the same amount of copper in their bones as is typical today. Therefore, any excess of copper in Roman bones above today's typical biologic level (received while living) would probably have come from moisture around burial artifacts, with *lead* undoubtedly being added from the same source at the same time.

We have in our Appendix B comparisons of copper with lead in bones from the following groups:

1. In an early (eneolithic) pre-Roman group of bones (found in Group D), we observe medians of about 7 ppm copper and 4 ppm lead, which might be considered minimally altered, or natural levels.

2. In the Roman poor we observe medians of about 25 ppm copper versus 35 ppm lead, which suggests some addition of soil copper and lead. However, these levels of both copper and lead are no more than twice those of modern

people today (who are so heavily exposed to industrial lead that they contain more than 100 times natural amounts[12]) so our observed uncorrected values for lead in the bones of the Roman poor are within a factor of two of the biologic lead level existing in them.

3. In the Roman rich we observe about 40 ppm copper versus 80 ppm lead. This definite excess of copper suggests that some of the lead in the bones of the rich came from burial artifacts. However, when Patterson considered this effect and estimated a correction for it (as he writes in Appendix A), he still found a large excess of lead in bones of the rich (150 ppm) compared to that in bones of the poor (40 ppm). (This difference is larger than that between the median values we have chosen to represent these two classes.) This indicates, we believe, that the differences between the rich and poor is biologic rather than coming from burial artifacts.

4. In Roman Emporion metal workers (Group A) we find 100 ppm copper versus 200 ppm lead. And in chemically altered Athenian bones from metallized well waters (Group E) we find about 320 ppm copper versus 340 ppm lead. The amounts of *copper* in these two groups of bones are clearly excessive, non-biologic, and originated from known associations with burial artifacts. Therefore, much of the excessive *lead* also probably came from burial artifacts.

It is easy to find defects in our procedures that lead to inaccuracies. But such defects could not overturn, nor seriously impugn our main thesis—that the ancient rich were for the most part so grievously leaded as to lower their effective fertility well below maintenance of their numbers, to damage their health and sanity, and often kill them. Constrastingly, most of the poor were not so badly afflicted that they were rendered infertile.

1. W. Specht & K. Fischer: Vergiftungsnachweis an den Resten einer 900 Jahre alten Leichen: *Archiv der Kriminologie*, 124:61, 1959.

2. See the note on page 104.

3. V. I. Prozorovsky & V. M. Kolosova: Some Spectrographic Studies on the Bone Tissue of Tsar Ivan IV, of his Sons and of Prince Skopin-Shuysky: *Sudebno Meditsinskaya Ekspertiza*, vol. 13, 2nd issue, April-June, 1970, pp. 7-11, with brief English summary. The Russian text was consulted.

4. Saul Jarcho: Lead in the Bones of Prehistoric Lead-glaze Potters: *Amer. Antiquity*, 30:94-6, 1964.

5. V. M. Kolosova & V. I. Pashkova, perhaps in the 1st vol., 1959, of *Sudebno Meditsinskaya Ekspertiza*, the Soviet Russian Jol. of forensic medicine.

6. See the note on page 107.

7. H. A. Schroeder & I. H. Tipton: The Human Body Burden of Lead: *Archives of Env. Health*, 17:965-78, 1968, Table 5.

8. D. P. Krause: Stable Lead in Human Bone: Argonne Natl. Lab., Radiological Physics Div., *Ann. Rept.*, Jan.-June 1961, pp. 77-80, Fig. 12.

9. Z. Jaworowski: *Stable and Radioactive Lead in Environment and Human Body*, Warsaw, 1967, 181 pp., p. 65, from vertebrae of 21 females.

10. H. P. Morris: Age and the Lead Content of Certain Human Bones: *Jol. of Indus. Hyg. & Toxicol.*, 22:100-3, graphing data from S. L. Tompset. A. B. Anderson, & G. Roche Lynch, Slater & Osler, From Morris' Figs. 2 & 3.

11. See the note on page 107.

12. C. Patterson. Contaminated and natural lead environments of man. *Archives of Env. Health*, 11:356 (1965).

9

Temporary Sterility Thru Heat

The Role of Clothing

That the ancient upper class males often became temporarily sterile thru too warm clothing and bathing, is probably a completely new idea, as applied to Rome. But our research makes it seem a reasonable supposition.

In the human species, as in most mammals, the testicles are in an exposed position. This would naturally make them cooler than the rest of the body. In most species (and perhaps in Nigerians[1] to a significant extent) this is further accentuated by lengthened, convoluted arteries to the testes, obviously to further cool the blood before it reaches those. Amelar[2] says the human testicles are in an environment normally cooler than within the abdomen by 2.2°C. Experiments with animals such as stallions and rams have shown that the warmth of an enclosing bag eliminated fertility. Harrison and Weiner[3] say, "If the heat is removed, a restoration of the sperm count back to normal may be seen within three months." Febril illness and *excessive alcohol* also depress the sperm count. Heinke and Doepfmer[4] cite cases of male infertility caused by supporters or by tight underwear, and cured by their abandonment. So do Simmons,[5] Hotchkiss,[6] and Cowles,[7] and we have ourself met a man cured of infertility by simply discarding his supporter, on medical advice.

The Roman male costume, at least in earlier times, provided next to the genitals a garment called a *subligaculum* (or *succinctorium, campestre,* Greek *perizoma,* later Latin *subligar),* of two alternative types, one like a modern supporter in front, in back only a strap passing between the buttocks; the alternative garment was a pair of drawers of half thigh length. Either form of *subligaculum*, but especially the first, the tighter one, might have been a factor for infertility. Atop the *subligaculum* the upper class man wore originally only the big, wrap-around, woolen toga. The common people used to sometimes wear a sort of cloak called a *cucullus*,[8] made of very coarse brown wool and provided with a hood. But in the third or second century B.C. the Roman gentlemen, following the Greeks and Etruscans, took to adding a tunic (Greek *chiton)* of wool or linen, a long shirt from neck to mid-thigh or as low as the ankle, and sometimes two of them in cold weather, or even more, between their toga and *subligaculum*. But often in warm weather the tunic was worn without a toga. Men working might omit either or both. "During the last century of the Republic and at the beginning of the Empire the toga became extremely wide and complicated (multifold), especially when it served as a ceremonial garment," says Boucher.[9] He cites Heuzey[10] who gives its layout as a segment of a circle, 5.6 meters on the chord and 2 m. across. Horace mocks a man whose toga was 2.66 m. wide. But in the second century A.D. the toga became more restricted; and later trousers were borrowed from the Germans. Smith et al[11] say that in Imperial times the *subligaculum* was chiefly confined to servants; but doubtless they were speaking of it as an only garment, as was often the case at work.

Another apparent instance (ancient but not Roman) of male sterilization by warm coverings, comes to us from the famous Greek physician Hippocrates[12] about 400 B.C. Describing the Sauromatae, Scythians living around the Sea of Azov, a region that had no grape products, he said they lived a pastoral life and that their ruling class were far and of low fertility: he claimed that as a result of such men riding horseback all day, with their legs hanging down, they developed varicose veins and became infertile and impotent. The ancients had neither saddles nor stirrups, but rode on a saddlecloth. If this were of thick wool, and likewise their trousers and perhaps further clothing, the combined and contained heats of horse and man might well have made them infertile.

All in all, we conclude that around the first century B.C. the costume of Roman gentlemen probably became too warm in the genital region for best fertility, and that the workers' costume did not. We infer that the gentlemen's costume became less sterilizing later, about the second century A.D.

The Role of Hot Bathing

It also appears fairly certain, as has been suggested by McNeill before us, that the ancients, especially their more idle men (who would presumably be richer on the average), suffered a considerable loss of fertility thru prolonged hot bathing.[13]   We have shown how clothing that overheats the testes, even a couple of degrees above normal, reduces male fertility temporarily but seriously. (Hot bathing has also been charged with inducing mutations, such as are practically always bad.)

Hot bathing seems to have begun in Greece, when her early centuries of rising wealth permitted such a luxury, in a land of scarce wood fuel. This custom, like so many others, was passed on to the Romans about the time of their conquest of Greece. Even the Greek language came to be used by the Roman aristocracy. Previous Roman bathing had been a harmless, private, bowl-and-pitcher affair, as Seneca tells.[14]   But Johnston says that after the Second Punic War (which ended in 292 B.C.), Romans began to build public heated baths like the Greek ones.[15]   Their number increased rapidly, at least 170 being operated in Rome alone in the year 83 B.C.; in time there were 952. With equal rapidity the hot baths spread thruout Italy and the provinces, till most towns and many villages had at least one. The greatest bath in Rome was that of Diocletian, which many of us have visited. These baths covered 12.5 hectares (31 acres) and included 1.36 ha. of pools. They could accommodate 3,600 bathers at once. Today the area contains a church, college, monastery, commercial building, the great circular Piazza della Repubblica, and the great National Museum of Archaeology (which has helped our researches with bones). Such bathing establishments rapidly spread to all the cities of the Empire. There were even baths for the private use of wealthy citizens.[14] Also hot springs were developed as spas, for example in Bath, England, where the water today is 45°C (113°F). The pool's bottom there was paved with lead, but that was probably unimportant.[15]

In 89 B.C. the "suspended bath" was invented: a wide fire-room some 65 cm. high,[16] topped by the masonry floor of a hot pool[17] *(caldarium)*, and usually having a sweat room too. Flues also warmed the walls of the building, like the hypocaust that came to heat the homes of the wealthy. Newly invented glass windows also illuminated without letting in cold drafts.

For the bathing there were various sequences, but most commonly the bathers passed from the sweat room or the hot pool to a *tepidarium* pool, thence to a cold pool and, after resuming their clothes, to a gymnasium and various facilities for recreation, eating and even culture.

Our chief points to notice are that the sweat room and the hot pool were very *hot.* In addition, altho the admission fee was minimal, the baths must have been most indulged in by those with the most leisure. We hear of some individuals spending all day at them. And we have quoted Seneca above, who wrote: "It makes no difference nowadays whether a bath is hot or on fire . . . We should condemn a slave found guilty of a crime to be washed alive." Again he speaks of "wanting to be cooked in one's bath," and calls the temperature of the sweat bath *(laconicum)* "like a fire."[14] Pliny[18] speaks of drunkards there "of whom the most cautious we see getting themselves cooked in hot baths from which they are carried away half dead." Farris[19] says "One feels that the practice of taking frequent hot baths has many commendable aspects; yet so common a diversion can, and often does, temporarily reduce the fertility of the man to the subfertile level."

Of course we have heard of hot baths in other countries too, such as the Turkish bath, the Finnish sauna in which the sweat bath is of fantastic temperature, and may be followed by a plunge in icy water or snow; and the Japanese hot baths and hot springs, very frequent and hot. Yet none of these peoples have died out nor suffered dysgenically, so far as we have heard. But such practices may well have reduced their natural fertility, and thereby substituted for other means of birth control, such as all countries have employed, including the Romans. And indeed, we have heard reports of the Japanese deliberately using the hot bath for birth control, but we have been unable to verify this.

Every additional factor tending to reduce births, whether conclusive, weak, or only occasionally effective, must by hypothesis reduce the growth rate of a stock (or speed its decimation). All we claim in this chapter is that over-warm clothing in the male genital region, and very hot bathing or sweat bathing by men, especially if long and frequent, must have reduced the Roman birthrate; and that such clothing and bathing were much more frequent among the rich than the poor, especially hot bathing among the *idle* rich who could spend long hours at it. This fits in with data from history, derived from ancient books and on tombstones: that the Roman rich after 150 B.C. had very few children, and dysgenically died out.

An apparently conforming case comes from the Havasupai Amerinds of Arizona,[20] who for a century maintained small families, averaging 4.2 people. Other methods of birth control were possible, but our author particularly noted that the men took four sweat baths an afternoon, at temperatures of 34-68°C (118-157°F), followed by plunges in an icy stream.

Once again *lead* apparently enters the picture. One symptom of lead poisoning is itching,[21] which may be painful. One's sweat contains the same proportion of lead as one's urine.[22] And bathing would alleviate the itch, I am assured by Detlev Stöfen.

We have spoken of the public baths of the cities, but there came to be also countless small, private baths in mansions both urban and rural. We can hardly imagine that these were used much by the slaves or poor people of the household or neighborhood, especially in view of the costliness of wood fuel, and the difficulties of ensuring a rural water supply. Next recall that there is a universal tendency for brains, in whatever rank of society, including slaves, to gravitate from the country to the cities, especially to the capitals. Furthermore, the rural mansion's bathing establishment, however comfortable and convenient, might not entice the gentleman to such long dalliance in it as would the great urban public establishments, with their spectacular architecture and abundant company, which often included women together with men in the later centuries.[23]

1. R. G. Harrison: Functional Importance of the Vascularization of the Testis, etc. in *Fertility and Sterility*, 3:366-75. On p. 369 he cites unpub. Nigerian data from R. M. Winston & H. G. Harrison.

2. Rich D. Amelar: *Infertility in Men*, 1944.

3. R. G. Harrison & O. S. Weiner: Abdomino-testicular temperature gradients: *Jol. Physiol.*, 107:48, 1948.

4. E. Heinke & R. Doepfmer, on pp. 8-10 of H. Schuermann & Doepfmer: *Fertilitätsstörungen beim Manne*, 1960, on p. 474.

5. F. A. Simmons: The Hypogonadal Male: *Fertility and Sterility*, 5:201-4, 1954.

6. R. S. Hotchkiss: *Fertility in Men*, 1944.

7. R. S. Cowles: Hypothermia, Aspermia, Mutation Rates and Evolution: *Qtly. Jol. of Biol,*, 40:356 etc., 1965.

8. Thos. Hope: *Costumes of the Greeks & Romans*, 1812-1962, p. 41.

9. F. L. L. Boucher: *Histoire du costume en occident*, Paris, Flammarion, 1965.

10. L. A. Heuzey: *Histoire du costume antique*, 1922, p. 238.

11. Wm. Smith & Waite & Marindin: *Dict. of Greek and Roman Antiquities*, article on *Subligaculum*.

12. Hippocrates: *On Airs, Waters and Places*, chapters 17-22.

13. Wm. H. McNeill: *The Rise of the West*, Univ. of Chgo. Press, 1963, p. 359, footnote 109.

14. Seneca, *Epistles*, 86:10.

15. H. W. Johnston: *Private Life of the Romans*, 1903, 344 pp., pp. 265-77.

16. Eduard Bäumer: *Geschichte des Badewesens*, 1903, 79 pp., Heft 7 of *Abhandlungen zur Geschichte der Medizin*, pp. 27 etc. Drawing of suspended bath on p. 27.

17. Wm. Gowland: Early Metallurgy of Silver and Lead, Part I, Lead,

in *Archaeologia*, 57:368-84, 1901.

18. Pliny,* 14:28.

19. Edm. J. Farris: *Human Fertility and Problems of the Male*, 211 pp., 1950, bib. on pp. 201-4, p. 11 cited.

20. Anita L. Alvarado: Cultural Determinants of Population Stability in the Havasupai Indians: *Am. Jol. Phys. Anthrop.*, 33:9-14, 1970.

21. U. S. Environ. Protection Agcy.: *Biological Aspects of Lead*, compiled by Irene R. Campbell & E. S. Meregard, an annotated bib. of lit. from 1950 thru 1964.
     Also Cantarow & Trumper,* p. 59.
     R. Fatzer: Anzeichen von Bleivergiftung?: *Schweiz. med. Wschr.*, 83:631-8, 1953. (Itching or stinging over the whole body is a symptom of lead poisoning.)

22. H. A. Waldron & D. Stöfen: *Sub-clinical Lead Poisoning*; Academic Press, Lon. & NY, 1974, p. 58.

23. Otto Kiefer: *Sexual Life in Ancient Rome*, Lon., Routledge & Kegan Paul, 6th impression, 1953, p. 158.

10

Social Forces

Celibacy

Celibacy in the Roman Empire was usually dysgenic. For it was probably practiced principally by an upper class far more concerned with its own pleasures or vices than with the welfare of the race. But celibacy can have various definitions. For present purposes the best definition would be non-marriage, especially if the goal was to avoid having children for whom one would be responsible. This, of course, does not imply an abstinence from sexual activity. Augustus, addressing an assemblage of men concerning his new *Jus trium liberorum* (granting privileges for fathers who produced three citizen children), said, "You are all having sexual relations."

Augustus realized that celibacy was dangerous for Rome. By the Julian laws he promulgated, celibates could not inherit unless they married within a hundred days of the death of the testator, nor could they attend public festivities or games. As with the Julian laws in general, these were commonly ignored; even Augustus admitted their failure when he repealed some later in his life. In later centuries the *Jus trium liberorum* came to be awarded even to childless men and bachelors.

It is difficult to establish when celibacy first became important in the Roman world, but it was known in the late Republic and became very common under the Empire. Vergil (70-19 B.C.) never married, and never seems to have felt the passion of Cupid's arrow. Perhaps he was the model for

Aeneas' character. For some time he occupied himself with a slave boy, but for most of his life he was known as "the virgin."[1]   But homosexuality was much less important among the Romans than the Greeks.

We suggest that lead poisoning had something to do with the prevalence of celibacy among patricians. For a great motive for marriage, in preference to irregular unions, was to obtain legal heirs. This was especially true in the earlier Republican days, when there were still patrician *gentes* to be continued. But when lead poisoning reduced the possibility of having children, why try to have them?

Religious Celibacy

Chaste celibacy, for religious or moral motives, was an idea old in the Far East. It first appeared in the Mediterranean world among the Essenes, a monastic sect of Jews in the second century B.C. (The Vestal Virgins at Rome we shall ignore, since they were so few.) The ideal of celibacy, akin to the Manichaean idea of the evilness of nature, arrived with the influx of the Manichaean and five other related religions and people from the Levant, as will be discussed in our following chapter. A like celibacy was present in another of those eastern cults, Mithraism, which numbered among its members virgins and other celibates. And there were a few homosexual and castration cults, such as that of Cybele. There are some inclinations toward religious celibacy in the New Testament, altho in his Epistles, St. Paul,[2] while suggesting celibacy as an ideal, demanded the right of clergy to marry. Marriage remained customary or frequent for all lower clerical ranks in Christianity, except among monastics, for 9 to 12 centuries, in much of western and always in eastern Europe.

The Romans regarded sexuality as a basic element in human life. In fact, we owe the word *sex* to them. Homosexuality was generally despised as "the Greek vice," and it was far less prevalent in Italy than in Hellas. Only one homosexual Roman emperor, Hadrian, died a natural death. The insane Elagabalus was assassinated when 17.

Birth Control

Tacitus assures us that contraception was common in Rome, and numerous ancient authors explain the methods to be used. According to Pike[3] sometimes sheaths of animal gut or of linen were used by either sex, as were pessaries of cyclamen root, cloth, or other materials, and suppositories chemically treated, often with lead salts (as we told in Chapter 3), or with oily or sticky substances. Yet the efficacy of these techniques, even when used by upper class people, is dubious. The poorer people, with less intelligence and money and no medical advisors, must have often used less effective, or worthless magical means, or none at all.

Hippocrates said that women should shake the sperm out of the vagina by jumping up and down after intercourse. Dioscorides recommended that root of brake or fern, or rennet of hare, be swallowed in an infusion, to cause miscarriage. The insertion into the womb of young shoots or leaves of ivy spread with honey was deemed effective. Soranus recommended that after every menstrual period women drink "water from the fire bucket of the smith." This might contain a little lead, to be sure. But far more effective and well known to the ancients were the rhythm method of timing intercourse (of course, without its recent Billings improvement), and the abnormal methods of coition, including withdrawal before ejaculation. The richer people, unwittingly, even had our latest favorite, oral contraception, in the form of leaded drinks. *Adynamon*, a favorite of courtesans, was one such drink, made by boiling down to half, doubtless in lead, a watered second squeezing of grapes, mixed with equal further water, or else evaporated. The oldest profession knew well they must avoid both pregnancy and much alcohol.

Various modern writers have studied ancient birth control, and Hopkins[4] considers that "the effect of contraception on Roman family limitation was negligible." But we cannot believe this in the face of all the above methods. Even if they did often fail, or fail to be generally used, they must have reduced the birthrate significantly, and especially in the upper, intelligent class, because we know that the birth

rate was low among them, and that several of their methods
were effective, often absolutely. But the poor, the ignorant,
and the weak-willed would naturally use them less, and less
skillfully, with no medical advisors, and with more readiness
to believe in the magical, unreliable methods.

Abortion

The frequent failure of contraception made abortion
and infanticide common ways of ending undesired pregnancies, or disposing of unwanted births. The demand for either
might arise as a result of poverty, family planning, or illegiti-
macy, with its denial of social status to the progeny of upper
class men from women of lower, or any but married status.
Balsdon comments: "In the late Republic and early Empire,
there were innumerable women of this sort, freedwomen for
the most part, elegant and attractive. These are the women
whom we have to thank for so much that is charming—and
indeed for not a little that is obscene—in Roman poetry."[5]
Pregnancies were often terminated in such cases. Ovid
wrote poems praying that his pregnant mistress Corinna
would survive an abortion. Juvenal wrote of the uncanny
skill of abortionists "paid to murder mankind within the
womb." Domitian was accused by his traducers of having
seduced his niece and then having forced her to undergo an
abortion, which killed her.

In an effort to protect the dying aristocracy against dilution by the new power elite that flooded Rome from the
Near East, Marcus Aurelius outlawed marriages between Senators and freedwomen. Other emperors imposed similar re-
strictions. The progeny of such affairs, many of which were
as stable and as much based on love as good marriages, had
little hope for their social future.[6]

What was the ancient attitude toward abortion? Aristotle not only refused to condemn it, but believed it should be
made obligatory once population had reached dangerous levels. Thruout the Roman Republic and into the early Empire,
no law banned it. But toward the end of the second century
Septimius Severus made abortion a crime. Ovid, Seneca,

Plutarch, and Juvenal all called abortion a criminal act, but all said it was a general practice. The first jurist to condemn it was Ulpian (d. 228 A.D.). The Christians from the outset took a posture of uncompromising hostility toward abortion. So as Christianity and its rival moralistic religious grew, so also did hostility toward abortion.

We know that some Roman wives went out in the streets during the *Lupercalia*, to be beaten with the leather strap which they hoped would make them fertile. We know that both Julius Caesar and Augustus wanted sons and were disappointed; we know that Nero and Domitian were saddened by the death of their children in infancy, and that Fronto, after losing five children in succession, cried out: "I never had a child born to me except when bereaved of another." Pliny wrote of the "misfortune" of a friend who was childless. The marriage of Scipio Africanus and Sempronia ended with no children and "so he hated her and she hated him." The higher the rank and wealth of a family, the more aristocratic its lineage, the more children (particularly sons) were felt a necessity.[7] Yet the higher the rank, the more the heirs were lacking. Why? Lead, *primum inter alia.*

Antiprogenitiveness

It is strange that we have to coin this new word, since the disposition it expresses has been practically universal in the human species, on frequent occasions in almost all if not every community and kind of people, ever since Homo sapiens acquired enough mind to think, plan, and act for his own or his fellows' welfare. For if nothing were done to check child production, the average woman might bear about a dozen children. And any man could beget a hundred or more. Such reproduction numbers are obviously too great, as an average, for any community, and would certainly be checked by starvation and many other consequences. We mention both this human potential of reproduction and the opposing desire for its limitation, because they were typical of the perishing Roman aristocracy.

Wealthy men without heirs in Roman times might be

courted by women who had either attractiveness or family connections to offer, and by young men hoping for an inheritance. Seneca comforted a mother who had lost her child by telling her, "with us childlessness gives more power than it takes away."[8] And Petronius, with habitual exaggeration, alleged "Crotona has only two classes of inhabitants, flatterers and flattered: and the sole crime there is to bring up children to inherit your money. It is like a battlefield at rest; nothing but corpses and the crows that pick them."[9] And this friend of Nero depicted Roman high society as one in which childbearing was avoided, so that the adults could in their old age enjoy the attention of flatterers eager to inherit their wealth.

But to believe that this was a general or even frequent motivation is, as Bálsdon[10] suggests, quite absurd. The childless adults had little reason to expect they would reach advanced age, given the Roman mortality rate. Nor should we suppose that many would prefer the calculated fawning of avaricious outsiders to the spontaneous affection of their own sons and daughters.

Infanticide

The practice of infanticide had long been a fact in ancient Rome. The Twelve Tables (IV:1) permitted a father to expose any deformed infant and any daughters after one. The Greeks had likewise practiced infanticide by exposure, as in the case of OEdipus. In the days of the Republic, M. I. Rostovtzeff[11] says, the patricians usually sought to limit the family size. If contraception or abortion did not work, then infanticide would, at least for girl babies. During the Republic the educated classes were the only ones who practiced it. Rostovtzeff says that the working class looked on children as an asset, to assist their parents in whatever occupation. This was especially true among farmers. In the large patrician class at least a son or two were necessary to continue the family name and the ancestor cult of the family *gens*. But after one or two sons were produced to secure those two purposes, few more children were desired.

In 445 B.C. the patricians, finding themselves without enough women of their class to marry, had obtained by the *Lex Canuleia* the right to marry plebeians. The shortage was a result probably not only of female infanticide, but also of the (recently proved) fact that the more masculine types of men, such as army officers, exact scientists, businessmen, and bald men, have about a third more sons than daughters; and vice versa.[12] Such men would naturally have more often obtained admission to the patrician class. Later, more efficient birth control methods probably replaced infanticide.

Whatever we may think of infanticide and the people who practiced it, the Romans arranged it as humanely as possible, exposing mainly deformed or sickly children, including doubtless some lead-poisoned ones. And the Roman method of infanticide by "exposure" was often not fatal. In Rome the exposure was usually at the base of the *Columna Lactaria* where the state provided wet nurses to save the babies. From there the unfortunate child might be adopted by a childless couple, or sold into slavery.[13] Thus as often happens today with unmarried mothers, a child was got rid of yet did not die, which appealed to ancient as to modern sentiment. But we cannot believe that they all survived. Some in Rome were abandoned not at the pillar in the Welabrum, a slum area, but at the edge of dung heaps or at open trenches used as sewers by the masses.

Suetonius tells of two outstanding teachers who had been abandoned as children. North African funerary inscriptions for foundlings of both sexes provide numerous references to their *educator, nutritor, patronus, patrona,* or foster parents, expressing gratitude for the kindness and love they received. In the first and second centuries A.D. foundations supported by such philanthropists as Pliny, cared for as many as 5,000 children of the poor, who might otherwise have died. And among the upper class there was great grief over children lost to disease (perhaps lead poisoning, so noxious to children).

---

12. Bernstein*: *Techniques.* The tendency is hereditary in the male line.

The exposure even of female children was discouraged by Augustus, and was illegal by the second century A.D. But the case was different with slaves, who probably comprised about half the population of the Eternal City. Here the issue was a coldblooded one of economics: whether to expose the female baby, and whether to make infertile one or both of her parents.[14] The two-to-one sex ratio in tomb inscriptions suggests that the impact of infanticide fell harder on females.

Abortion and exposure (infanticide) must have been especially common when the parentage crossed established class lines, or was illegitimate. Indirect evidence of this is the infrequence of references to illegitimate children, until the third century. This condition changed only with the democratization of the Empire, and with religious change, which tended both to respect all lives, and to break down class separations, and hence to increase the scope of potentially legitimate unions. In order to raise more revenues by imposing death duties and slave manumission taxes on citizens, Caracalla extended the privilege of Roman citizenship to all his free subjects. Soon thereafter there were in essence only two great free classes in the Empire: the *honestiores*, comprising landowners, officers, officials and town councillors, and the *humiliores*, comprising everyone else but slaves. The *humiliores* were bound to their trades or to the soil, could be flogged, tortured or summarily put to death, rather like slaves.[15]

The system of Diocletian transformed Rome into more of a totalitarian state than Persia had ever been. Equality was approached by leveling downward. And bastardy became more familiar, of which anon.

Enforced Sterility

In the immense slave populations sterility was oftenest enforced by separation of the sexes. Castration was little used, but infibulation was often imposed to make fertile intercourse impossible. With women slaves this was accomplished by a piercing brooch across the vagina: for men, by a metal disk around the end of the penis. In great mansions of the richest there might be a hundred or more slaves; and especially in rural estates and in mines or quarries, large numbers made enforced segregation fairly easy. So in the large plantations, and especially in the death traps of the mines and quarries, enforced sterility carried a racial bias, since to these occupations were assigned the slaves captured in war, especially the northern barbarians. They were big, strong, uncouth people, speaking languages no one could understand, and were thot useful only for agricultural or industrial labors.

In contrast the native-born or the Levantine slaves were civilized people, and spoke Greek or some other language that could be understood, so they were usable for household slaves or in industry, or even as clerks or teachers. Thus they might please their masters, be allowed offspring or made concubines, and were very often freed after long and faithful service. Thus they would contribute to the Roman race, culture, and religion, as we shall tell in our next chapter about the Levantine influx. But the many captured barbarian slaves, or Nordic or Alpine race, who might have transformed and perhaps improved the Roman race, were mostly segregated, childless, and often worked to death.

Venereal Disease

Venereal disease has been suspected as a cause for a declining population among the Romans, but may be quickly eliminated from the list of likely suspects. Whatever the date of origin of syphilis (a complicated and much disputed issue), there is an informed consensus that it did not exist in the ancient world in its modern or in any serious form. The possibility of a venereal disease that was unimportant, as some have reported, is shown by the fact that we recognize six venereal diseases today, of which only two are important. The infectious diseases are constantly changing, as we know from the ever new varieties of influenza, partly thru the resistance acquired by their hosts, and much more by the evolution of their own powers of attack, thru their far more frequent generations.

The case against gonorrhea, the only other modern

venereal disease that could cause sterility, is more complicated.   Ronald Hare wrote in an authoritative survey of ancient diseases that gonorrhea was "well known to the Romans."[16] He was probably misled in this matter by the fact
that the word gonorrhea, meaning "a flow of seed," was
coined by Galen (ca. 130 A.D.). However, as Garston and
Thayer point out (as reported by Dubois): Galen's own definition and description of gonorrhea is equivalent to what
today is termed spermatorrhea."[17]   In fact, the first clear
reference to gonorrhea that shows awareness of its venereal
origin is by Guillaume de Sallice in the thirteenth century.

Bastardy

Bastardy occurred chiefly from an unsanctioned connection between a man of higher and a female of lower class,
in spite of birth control, abortion, and infanticide. The lower
the woman's rank, the less the likelihood that she would be
sterilized by lead, or her child killed by it, or that birth control would be effective. We hardly ever hear of bastards in
Roman times, until the third century A.D. Tho they were
doubtless numerous, parentage must have been kept secret.
Bastardy was not acceptable among the Romans until a late
date. This is in notable contrast to its treatment in medieval
times.

The emperor Constantius may have been a bastard of
Claudius Gothicus, emperor in 268 to 270 A.D. His son by a
concubine, Helena, became Constantine the Great. He in
turn produced Crispus, an illegitimate son by his concubine,
and had him murdered. Said Balsdon, "No great stigma attached to being a concubine's child."[18]

Still concubinage and bastardy never became widespread and respectable among the upper classes of Rome,
even in the last centuries of the Western Empire. In contrast,
in medieval Europe illegitimate children were given a recognized place in the social order. Before his successes in sub-
duing Normandy and conquering England, William the Con-
queror was known as William the Bastard. The surname Fitz-
roy, meaning son of the king, was applied to the illegitimate

sons of a sovereign. As late as the reign of Victoria, the bastard children of her grandfather and uncles were ennobled, received at court, and given command of armies and government of colonies. But in Roman times no bastard could expect any public acceptance by virtue of high but illegitimate paternity.

As the Roman Empire gradually froze into the stifling rigidities of Diocletian's system, abortion and infanticide may have become more widespread. Rostovtzeff concluded that "race suicide was typical of the age," adding that it was "favored by Roman legislation concerning the exposure of infants and abortion." He found preponderant evidence that very few families either of the upper or of the lower classes cared to rear children."[19] (But of course children do not have to be wanted to be born and raised.)

Assortative Mating

Francis Galton, the brilliant cousin of Darwin and father of Eugenics, observed that English peerages were continually being extinguished. When the distinguished Roman scholar Hugh Last read this passage and R. A. Fisher's comment on it,[20] it occurred to him that Galton's insight might be applicable to Roman society.[21] Studies of domestic animals prove that reduced fertility is hereditary, Galton said. He continued: "Consequently the issue of a peer's marriage with an heiress frequently fails and his title is brot to an end."[22] But no one seems to have taken up this study in the several decades since Last's remark.

Yet here is an opportunity for an additional understanding of not only Roman but all advanced countries. Last's remark is one illustration of assortative mating, people marrying their own kind, which Jensen and Eckland[23] have pointed out as a great basis for evolution, whether up-

20. A noble heiress is one who had no surviving brother, and perhaps no sisters either, therefore likely from an infertile stock. R. A. Fisher: *Genetic Theory of Natural Selection.* (Oxford U. Press, 1930.)

ward or downward. Jensen showed that assortative mating
produces eighty percent of the I.Q.'s above 145.

Civil Wars Followed by Proscriptions

The sad history of civil wars, and their far greater frequency in the later years of the Empire, afford striking evidence of the decline of intelligence in the Roman ruling class.
From about 509 B.C., when the last Etruscan king was ex-
pelled and a Republic set up guaranteeing leadership to the
patrician class, there occurred *not one civil war* for about 420
years, until the aristocrat Sulla in 87 B.C. rebelled against the
popular party of the illiterate Marius, ending more than four
centuries of domestic peace. What other country, for instance our own, could boast of such a record of freedom
from civil war?

Thereafter followed a period of frequent civil wars,
headed by Marius, Pompey, Cicero, Crassus, Caesar et al, until Octavian vanquished Antony at Actium in 29 B.C., ending
a 69-year epoch of frequent civil wars. Octavian was then able
to consolidate his power and set up a cult of near worship of
the emperor, now renamed Augustus. And tho he had no
son, only a daughter, he was able to bequeath the throne to
his stepson Tiberius, who in turn found a relative in Caligula,
who was manifestly insane (likely from lead). He in turn had
an uncle, Claudius, to leave the throne to, and Claudius was
able to find and prepare a relative to succeed him before he
was poisoned, namely Nero, who reigned from A.D. 54 to 68.
Nero did not fiddle while Rome burned (the fiddle had not
been invented), but his follies were more than enough to
bring revolt and his suicide. This left no possible successor of
the Julian *gens;* so there ensued a civil war between four
generals, of whom Vespasian was the winner. He was succeeded by his own sons in succession, Titus and Domitian, and on
the latter's murder, by the elderly Nerva. Tho he reigned
little more than a year, dying in 98, he was able to establish a
good system of succession, that of each emperor *adopting* a
grown man of proved ability to be his colleague in government and ultimately his heir. Called the Antonine succession,

it was the perfect solution for a situation in which people like emperors would probably have no legitimate sons, and democracy was impossible. The system worked well for a century, thru the reigns of Trajan, Hadrian, Antoninus Pius, and Marcus Aurelius. But Aurelius' wife, Faustina, the daughter of Antoninus, bore him 11 (or 13) children, of whom four still survived when he died at age 59. Unfortunately under political pressure he appointed one of them, Commodus, to be his successor. But when only 19 years old, Commodus was attacked, became tryannical, and was successfully assassinated in A.D. 191, after 13 years of rule.

After each civil war the winning party was likely to proscribe and kill the *leaders* of the defeated party. Yet, to be sure, these proscriptions, tho killing the better men, the leaders, were not so harmful to the race as they might seem, for the leaders who were killed were commonly older, leaded men with wives in the same leaden pickle, from whom one would not expect many more children to be born and survive anyway. Yet with the extremely frequent divorces a leader might well have had a younger wife; or he might yet beget a son by some mistress or slave, who if he lived, would carry on half of his father's genes, tho probably not his name or all of his culture.

In the case of Maximinus Thrax, a shepherd of enormous height and strength, who rose to be emperor in 235-8 A.D., he perpetrated not only proscriptions, but in Africa and Italy massacres of the upper class.[24]

In any case civil wars, and proscriptions of leaders, are certainly bad for any country economically, culturally, and genetically. And it is evident that those ever-recurrent civil wars, from Sulla's revolt in 87 B.C., and especially after the assassination of Commodus in 192 A.D., onward (and downward) to the traditional end of the Empire in 476 A.D., were bad for the race, ruinous for civilization as well as empire, and must have been largely caused by lead poisoning and other dysgenic genocultural forces, which deprived emperors of male heirs. Caracalla killed 20,000 people about 212 A.D. Elagabalus was obviously insane and was soon killed. After Maximinus' assassination in 238 there were 26 recognized emperors in fifty years, or 48 from Commodus' murder to the end of the Empire, each emperor reigning an average of 5.9 years. These statistics suggest much about the intelligence of the then upper class, and about their continuing destruction, by lead and other dysgenic factors.

Moreover, these assassinations, civil wars, and proscriptions were written on the papyrus of ancient history by their old *lead* pencil. For lead poisoning certainly could have played a major part in the follies of emperors and of their rival assassins and proscribers. One would suspect some plumbism from the perfidy of their actions, since some outstanding symptoms of plumbism are violence, aggressiveness, impulsiveness, hyperactivity and insanity. D. Bryce-Smith and H. A. Waldron,[25] Detlev Stöfen, and many others have pointed this out.

Summary

If we attempt to add up the net effect of our ten social factors that remolded the Roman race and culture, we conclude that they were pervasive and powerful dispensers of life and death; yet we often cannot speak positively about what qualities they bred into or out of the Roman race. If we evaluate these ten social forces in the order of their consideration above, we think that celibacy, especially if religious, was dysgenic; birth control, dysgenic; abortion, probably so; antiprogenitiveness, a question; infanticide, eugenic; enforced sterility, dysgenic; venereal disease, unimportant; bastardy, eugenic; assortative mating, a question; and the proscriptions following civil wars, dysgenic.

If we should add these factors up we get five dysgenic, two eugenic, and three doubtful or unimportant. On the whole these social factors seem to have weighed on the downward side, against the elevator of the human race, the survival of the fittest.

1. Suetonius: *On Poets*, Loeb ed., Vergil, p. 9.
2. I Corinthians 7:32. But cf. 7:25 and 9:5; also I Timothy 3:1, 12; and Titus 1:6.

3. E. Roylston Pike: *Love in Ancient Rome*, (Lon., Muller, 1965), pp. 235, 242.

4. Keith Hopkins: Contraception in the Roman Empire: *Comparative Studies in Society and History*, 1965, 6, p. 142.

5. J. P. V. D. Balsdon: *Roman Women*, (Lon., Bodley Head, 1962), p. 233.

6. R. Syme: Bastards in the Roman Aristocracy, *Proc. of Am. Philos. Soc.*, 1960, pp. 323-7.

7. J. P. V. D. Balsdon: *Life and Leisure in Ancient Rome*, (NY, McGraw-Hill, 1969), pp. 84-87.

8. Seneca: *Ad Marciam*, XIX, 2.

9. Petronius: *Nero*, (Henderson ed.), p. 326.

10. Baldsdon, *Life and Leisure in Ancient Rome*, supra.

11. M. I. Rostovtzeff: *Social and Econ. Hist. of the Roman Empire*, (Lon., Oxford U. Press, 2nd ed., 1957), vol. 1, p. 476.

12. Bernstein,* The tendency is hereditary in the male line.

13. Pike, supra, p. 242.

14. C. D. Darlington: *The Evolution of Man and Society*, (NY, Simon & Schuster, 1969), p. 275.

15. Michael Grant: *The Climax of Rome*, (Boston, Little Brown, 1968), p. 83.

16. Ronald Hare: *The Antiquity of Diseases Caused by Bacteria and Viruses*, a Review of the problem from the Bacteriologist's Point of View, in Don Brothwell and A. T. Sandison, eds.: *Diseases of Antiquity*, (Springfield, Chas. C. Thomas pub., 1967), p. 128.

17. R. W. Dubois: *Bacterial and Mycotic Infections of Man*, 3rd ed., 1958, p. 505.

18. Balsdon, *Roman Women*, supra, p. 233.

19. Rostovtzeff, supra, p. 476.

20. See the note on page 131.

21. Hugh Last: Letter to N. H. Baynes, in *Jol. of Roman Studies*, 1947, pp. 152-6.

22. Francis Galton: *Hereditary Genius*, 1869, (Cleveland, World, 1962), pp. 178-9.

23. Bruce K. Eckland: Evolutionary Consequences of Differential Fertility and Assortative Mating in Man: *Evolutionary Biology*, 5: 293-305, 1972. Page 301 cites p. 36 of A. R. Jensen's famous 1969 article How Much Can We Boost IQ?: *Harvard Educ. Rev.*, 39:1-123.

24. S. Mazzarino: *End of the Ancient World*, tr. by Geo. Holmes, pp. 155 ff.

25. Cf. D. Bryce-Smith & H. A. Waldron: Lead, Behavior and Criminality: *Ecologist*, 4:367-77, 1974; and our Chapter 8.

11

Population Decline
and the Levantine Influx

There is a consensus of scholars that a significant and serious decline in the Empire's population probably occurred during the early centuries of the Christian era, most massively from the third century onward. Whatever its extent and causes, there is some relation of this decline to our thesis on the decline of quality and culture in the population. For lead poisoning affected the poor as well as the rich, tho not so much. And a smaller and sicker population (if other things were equal or worse) would naturally reduce the number of inventors and therefore inventions. We shall cite in our next chapter Darmstaedter's data[1] showing a much worse decline of the frequency of inventions and discoveries, to 6.75 percent, comparing the first century A.D. with the fifth. Why is the modern world turning out inventions so much faster than in Roman times? Well, in answer, why did New York State citizens take three times the patents won by Massachusetts citizens in the same years? Obviously because New York had three times the population, being otherwise similar.[2]

The population of Roman cities has been gaged by changes in their areas, proved from the contraction of their walls. It is estimated that when the Gallic cities were refortified against renewed Germanic invasions in the third century, their area had shrunk to a fourth or an eighth of their first century extent. Yet a continual influx of barbarian agricultural settlers *(laeti)* and military allies *(foederati),* from the time of Marcus Aurelius' Marcomannic wars onward, suggests that farm land was always available for new settlers. Barbarians were imported *en masse* by Marcus Aurelius, Valentinian, Aurelian, Probus, and Constantine, from the mid-second to the early fourth century. So many farms had been abandoned in Italy (perhaps from climatic change[3] and/or soil exhaustion[4]) that Pertinax (emperor 193 A.D.) offered farms gratis to anyone who would cultivate them.[5]

In his monumental work on the sconomic and social history of the Roman Empire, M. I. Rostovtzeff stressed the depopulation of Greece and Italy as major causes and symptoms of their decay. He argued that Trajan's wars contributed to Italy's loss of people and crops.[6] Hence Domitian tried to save the peninsula by prohibiting competitive vineyards in the provinces, Nerva redistributed Italian acreage to the poor and Trajan settled veterans near Rome, and prohibited emigration from Italy.

Along with the loss of population in Italy, we observe a wider scattering of the Empire's leadership. And the capitals or centers of leadership moved farther north, perhaps partly because of climatic change, and the coming of malaria, and also in accord with Gilfillan's law of Coldward Progress while civilization advances.[7] So Milan, Aquileia (near Venice), Lyons and even Trier became prominent, and of course Constantinople. The Senate was no longer filled primarily with Italians, and after the Antonine succession of adopted emperors ended with Marcus Aurelius, only a few of the Empire's chiefs were of Italian origin. Greek largely replaced Latin as the preferred language of the ruling class. Among emperors, Diocletian had begun life as a Dalmatian slave, Constantine was the illegitimate son of an innkeeper, and Justinian was an Illyrian barbarian, tho with a good Greek education. His wife was from the lowest profession.

Otto Seeck, in a voluminous and oft-cited history of the ruin of the ancient world,[8] stressed the *Ausröttung der besten*, the extermination of the best. But not knowing

---

7.   S. C. Gilfillan: The Coldward Course of Progress; *Pol. Sci. Qly.*, 35:393-410, 1920, and in *Historical Outlook*, 12:8-15, 1921. Also see Appendix D.

about lead poisoning (nor possible heat influences) he was unable to influence egalitarian thinkers.

As Greece is usually our prototype for Rome, so after Greece's more catastrophic decline of genius, we find a comparable decline of population. A late Greek-language historian, probably Pausanias of the second century A.D., in telling of the host of soldiers the fifth century B.C. Greeks had gathered to repulse the Persian invasion, said that in his own day they could hardly produce one-tenth that many.

In the Dark Ages (after 476), still further depopulation occurred. And lead poisoning appears in some of our Group D bones assayed from that period, in Appendix B.

Decline in Wealth

Along with a decline in population went a similar decline in wealth. Zabinski[9] has shown that the wages of agricultural laborers in the time of Diocletian were only sufficient to buy 1.29 standard life-sustaining rations, and that of a stone-cutter only enough for 2.58 such. These wages were "clearly insufficient for maintaining a family" and were definitely inferior to the wages prevailing in Greece in the fourth century B.C. Such an inability to support families would naturally cause a further decline in population.

Census Data

Ancient Roman population data are very incomplete and unreliable, especially in terms of age, sex, occupation, social class, ethnic origin, and region. One reason is that the classical world was habitually careless in its use of quantitative data. The Greek and Latin numerical system made the manipulation of large numbers cumbersome, even with their abacus, which with its successive rods or lines did embody the principle of decimal place value. The ancients' difficulty with large numbers is reflected in the fact that the Greek word *myriad* meant both 10,000 and any number so large as to be almost inconceivable. Had the ancients possessed the decimal system of written notation they would have left us with more accurate statistics.[10]

Paradoxically Rome gave the world the word *census,* yet Roman population remains an enigma. Every five years, the Roman Republic counted its members and their property. The population count was extended by Augustus to cover the whole Empire. And this was continued until Vespasian's reign (69 A.D.). Yet we do not even know whether women were included, nor what areas were covered.[11] All modern estimates of the empire's population take as their starting point Julius Beloch's classical study, now almost a century old.[12] He estimated the population at 54 million at the death of Augustus in 14 B.C., of whom 11.5 million were in Africa, 6.6 million in Italy and Sicily, 6 million in Iberia, and 3 million in Greece. More recent studies have revised these estimates upward.

In the sparse ancient census data we have found only two bits of information on the number of children present. In a study by Michel (cited by Landry)[13] of the census inscriptions, from probably a better district of Troy in the Hellenistic age, reported for 136 men that 65 percent were celibate; among the married, 54 percent were childless, 28 percent 2 children, and 6 percent 3 children. (In France in 1926, when population was decreasing, only 23 percent were celibate.) Of course a celibate man might be begetting bastard children, but they would not inherit upper-class rank, wealth, power nor education, and probably only half of upper-class genes. The other inscription from an apparently good district of Miletus, between the third and first centuries B.C., allows us to conclude that naturalized men, probably an oldish group, had but 1.36 children per man.

Life Expectancy

Another line of evidence is from Dr. J. L. Angel's[14] examination of the age at death of skulls found in various parts of Greece, whose owners had enough rank to be buried

10.   Our so-called Arabic number system, regularizing place value, was devised in India, probably in the 7th century A.D., and spread to the West by 769, thru the Arabs.

in cemeteries. He found their life span improving from the prehistoric to the classical period (650—150 B.C.), from 35 to 38 years on average, then declining thru the Roman period (males 42 years, females 31.6) to the Byzantine figure of 33.7.   Again, data from an Egyptian census of A.D. 175 showed an expectation of life at birth of something less than 27 years.

Writings attributed to the jurist Ulpian, from the second and third centuries A.D., provide a table of life expectancies, probably not covering the lower classes, since it was for use in law suits. For ages up to 20 he accorded a 30-year expectation of life, decreasing to 27 years at ages 20-25, 13 at ages 46-47, 9 at ages 50-55, and 5 when over 60 years.[15]

Epigraphic Evidence of Life Span

Epigraphy is the study of carved inscriptions, which for our purposes are all on tombstones, save for the two pieces of census data, from Roman Troy and from Miletus reported above from Landry.   But the tombstones have a marked limitation in that they cover primarily the middle and lower middle classes.[16]   The vast mass of the poor are underrepresented, as are the very rich.   This reduces epigraphy's value for testing our main thesis. The tombstone records seem to indicate that the rich lived longer than the poor.   But the poor had many causes for death beside lead poisoning, notably poverty, and lack of physicians. Furthermore a child would not be apt to have a tombstone telling his age.

Another limitation of epigraphy is that recording of birth and death dates, or of age, did not become general until the reign of Tiberius (14-37 A.D.). As Kajanto has pointed out, the recording of infant mortality is very incomplete, and the older age groups are overrepresented in indications of age.[17]

Still, based on a study of over 30,000 funerary inscriptions, J. C. Russell[18] estimated that in the city of Rome life expectancy at birth was only 15.3 years for males and 16.3 for females. In Latium it was even lower, but in all other parts of the Empire higher, up to 29 years in Egypt if the data can be trusted. (The city of Rome probably had an unusual number of young immigrants.)

A. R. Burn[19] reassessed Russell's data, to calculate the remaining expectancy for those who had survived to age 15. He found this shockingly short, even worse than in India in 1901. In Roman Britain half of those who survived to age 15 would be dead at 37, in Spain at 36, in the Danube area at 33, and in an African military settlement at 38. Durand[20] concluded that infant mortality may have carried off 30 to 40 percent of Roman neonates (suggestive of lead poisoning). At this rate women would have had to average five children to sustain a slow rate of population increase.

Burn's[21] North African data showed that the average life span for males surviving to age 15 was to 38, for 447 slaves and freedmen of Carthage, to 45 for 616 members of a middle class group, and to 48 for 442 residents of upper-class districts. So the life span spread between rich and poor was ten years in these first and second-century groups. A much later sample, of 210 Christian males in the fourth to sixth centuries, showed an average life span of 52 years. From this Burn inferred that health improved during the period. But a much likelier inference would be that the Christian group was simply richer than any of the three earlier pagan communities. If so, the indicated difference of life span between very rich and moderately poor was 14 years in favor of wealth.[22] This striking spread indicates that the biological extinction of the upper classes required massive impairment of their fertility, since their death rate would not explain it.

The Fertility of the Aristocracy

The eminent historian of the Roman Empire, Tenney Frank[23] analyzed the fertility of patrician families. He found that of 400 families of Senators in 65 A.D., half had become extinct 31 years later. Of 45 noble families in the time of Caesar only one, the Cornelii, still existed in 117 A.D. These two rates of decline are compatible, since the second period was five times as long as the first. The implication is that the average aristocratic couple produced only one surviving child. In other words, the patrician death rate was about double their effective, surviving birthrate. Surely there must have been potent aristocidal factors, such as lead poisoning.

There was an extraordinary frequency of divorce among the aristocracy. But we do not think this would have lowered the legitimate birthrate. Rather it was an *indication* of a low birthrate. For if a couple had living children they would be more apt to stick together. Such matters, especially the great frequency of celibacy, have been briefly discussed in our previous chapter.

Augustus made futile efforts to save the ever perishing aristocracy, as we have told. Dio Cassius observed[24] "And since among the nobility there were far more males than females, he allowed all free men who wished (except Senators) to marry freedwomen, and ordered that their offspring be held legitimate." We doubt the male surplus was caused by female infanticide, but rather by the observed higher death rate of ancient women (probably from childbearing difficulties). In addition Marianne Bernstein* has used statistics to prove that the more masculine type of men, such as army officers, lawyers, business leaders, engineers, and physical scientists (except chemists), are not only often bald (an almost exclusively male trait) but have more sons than daughters, by a margin of around 35 percent. We have pointed this out in Chapter 10, and have confirmed it by abundant personal observation. Since the masterful masculine type would naturally predominate among those who had scrambled to the top in Roman society, they would beget considerably fewer daughters than sons.

Comparison of Noble Fertility of Rome versus Later Europe

We have guessed that the average Roman aristocratic couple in the time of Augustus produced only about one surviving child, tho the wife may have had several pregnancies. How does this compare with the fertility of the top class in other periods? Sigismund Fuller's study of the births and deaths of 2,888 male members of European ruling families between 1500 and 1925, provides a revealing comparison.[25]

During the sixteenth century these men begot an average of 6.8 children; during the seventeenth, 7.1 children; in the eighteenth, 5.8 children; and in the nineteenth, 4.9. Even in the first quarter of the present century such men fathered on the average 3.2 offspring.

Thus we see a very sharp contrast between the reproductive performance of later European royalty, and that of the Roman aristocracy. The contrast suggests either a voluntary abstention of the Roman elite, or far more likely, their sterilization by forces over which they had no control. But a combination of both would be likely. Thus the demographic data from Rome reenforce our hypothesis that lead poisoning, and probably localized heat and other factors we have noted, were the greatest causes of Rome's catastrophic genetic, cultural, and political declines.

The Levantine Influx

There is abundant evidence that during our period the western Roman world, and particularly the cities of Italy, were being flooded by people from eastern ethnic and cultural backgrounds. Juvenal said that nowadays the Orontes (the river of Damascus) flows into the Tiber. Thruout the second century the ranks of the middle (and therefore ultimately the upper) classes were thus gradually pervaded by eastern people, whose acculturation to Roman traditions was by no means thoroly effected. Some came as free migrants, others as slaves. Those from the Near East who had been enslaved were not often captives in war, but had been kidnapped as poor men, or sold as youths by poor parents into what might be a better life. In any case they were civilized people and spoke some language known among household slaves or other Orientals. If they knew some Greek, their chances were best, since Greek became the second and more elegant language of the Roman aristocracy. So Levantine slaves or freedmen could fit into a Roman community, produce children legitimate or otherwise, and have a good chance of manumission some day if they served well. In contrast, the slaves captured on the western and northern frontiers were uncouth barbarians, who spoke incomprehensible Iberian, Celtic, Ger-

manic, or Slavic tongues. Such slaves were employed mainly
as gang laborers on rural estates, or in the quarries or mines,
and were allowed little chance for reproduction. Life was
hard and short for them, so they had little of the transform-
ing impact on Roman culture that the Levantine slaves had.

Tenney Frank,[26] from his study of 13,900 sepulchral
inscriptions, showed the magnitude of the Levantine influx.
He concluded from names and from the frequent "L" for
Libertus (freedman) that the West was inundated by Greek
and Oriental slaves. He estimated that ultimately ninety percent of the capital city's inhabitants were of foreign extrac-
tion, and that this accounted not only for religious change
but, as he thot, for the familiar decline.

The Levantine influence became most clearly operative in the field of religion, by the introduction of *six* somewhat similar religions from the same region. There came,
thru immigrants and converts, not only Christianity, but Jud-
aism, Mithraism, the Samaritan religion, Marcionism (a rebel
sect of Christianity); and Manichaeanism, to which St. Augus-
tine once belonged. This last religion later resurfaced in the
Bogomils of the Balkans and the Albigensians of Aquitaine.
Notable among these Levantine religions was Mithraism, to
which Christianity owes the change of Christmas from Janu-
ary 6 (Twelfth Night, Epiphany) to December 25, Mithras
Day, near the winter solstice, and perhaps also the change
from the Sabbath to Sun-day, and perhaps the halo. All of
these Levantine religions were monotheistic, and also dualis-
tic (God versus Satan, good versus evil, light versus darkness,
spiritual versus worldly, heaven versus hell); and all were
moralistic, and had a certain egalitarian, middle-class flavor,
contrasting with the aristocratic nature of the old paganism.
The numerous Gnostic sects were also involved with this
group of eastern religions, especially with Christianity and
Marcionism.

Another novel element, related to the moralistic emphasis of these eastern religions, was asceticism. Most took a
skeptical view of the pleasures of the flesh, especially the
Mithraic religion, which had some celibates. We have spoken
of this in our previous chapter concerning religious celibacy.

1. P. Sorokin: *Social and Cultural Dynamics*, vol. II, utilizing Darmstaedter's count of inventions by century.
2. Gilfillan: *Supplement to the Sociology of Invention*. (San Francisco Press, 1971), Principle 22 on pp. 35-7; and Chapter 4B on Inventiveness by Nation & Race, and pp. 163-71 on Why the Classical Age was Uninventive. Or the same briefly in *Technology and Culture*, 3:85-7, 1962.
3 Columella,* XII:39, 42.
4. V. Simkhovich: Hay and History: *Pol. Sci. Qtly.*, 28:3-31, 1913.
5. Will Durant: *Caesar and Christ*, 1944, p. 368.
6. M. I. Rostovtzeff: *Social and Econ. Hist. of the Roman Empire*. (Oxford, Clarendon Press, 1963), I:358.
7. See the note on page 137.
8. Otto Seeck: *Geschichte des Untergangs der antiken Welt*, 1921, 6 vols.
9. Z. Zabinski: The Biological Index of the Buying Power of Money, in Robt. Forster & O. Ranum, eds.: *Biology of Man in History: Selections from the Annales*, (Balto., Johns Hopkins U.), p. 186.
10. See the note on page 139
11. T. H. Hollingsworth: *Historical Demography*, (Cornell U. Press, 1969), p. 69.
12. K. Julius Beloch: *die Bevölkerung der griechisch-römischen Welt*, 1886.
13. A. Landry: Qq. aperçus concernant la dépopulation dans l'Antiquité Gréco-romaine; in *Rev. Historique*, 177:1-33, 1936, pp. 2-3. citing on Troy Ch. Michel: *Recueil d'inscriptions Grecques*, No. 667; and on Miletus Wiegand: *Milet, Ergebnisse*, Bd. 1, Heft 3, pp. 55-105.
14. J. L. Angel: Length of Life in Ancient Greece: *Jol. of Gerontol.*, 2:18, Jan. 1947.
15. Josiah C. Russell: Late Ancient and Medieval Population: *Trans. of Amer. Philos. Soc.*, ser. 2, vol. 48, part 3, 1958, p. 24.
16. A. R. Burn: Hic Breve Vivitur: *Past and Present*, IV:2-31, 1953.
17. I. Kajanto: *On the Problem of the Average Duration of Life in the Roman Empire*, Helsinki, 1968.
18. Russell, supra, pp. 25-59.
19. Burn, supra.
20. Jn. D. Durand: Mortality Estimates from Roman Tombstone Inscriptions: *Amer. Jol. of Sociology*, 65:365-73, 1960.
21. Burn, supra.
22. Kajanto, supra.
23. Tenney Frank: Race Mixture in the Roman Empire: *Amer. Hist. Rev.*, 21:253-4, 1916.

24. Dio Cassius: *Roman History*, LIV:16.
25. Sigismund Fuller: Births and Deaths among Europe's Ruling Families since 1500; in D. V. Glass & D. E. C. Eversley, eds., *Population in History*, (Chgo., Aldine, 1965), pp. 87-100
26. Tenney, supra, p. 705 etc.

12

Decline of Genius and Culture

Appraisals of culture and civilization are necessarily to some degree arbitrary and subjective. Still, there are periods in history that are considered, in the consensus of those competent to judge, to be ages of high creativity, while others are deemed ages of stagnation or decline. The decay of Roman culture and civilization after the death of Marcus Aurelius was so precipitous and general that one could not find a competent scholar who would question the decadence.

In the context of this book, Roman culture means the intellectual achievements of the leading inhabitants of the Roman Republic or Empire, whether Italian, Spanish, Greek, Egyptian, or of any other nationality, and regardless of whether they wrote in Latin or in Greek. The requirement for inclusion is merely that they were subjects of Rome.

The period of our consideration stretches from 150 B.C., marking the Roman conquest of Greece (and the Greek intellectual conquest of Rome) to 476 A.D., when Romulus Augustulus, the last emperor in the West, was deposed by barbarian mercenaries led by Odoacer. During parts of this period Egypt, Syria, and Palestine were independent of Rome. Nevertheless, we have thot of the Roman Empire as including all lands west of Persia.

The mainly lead-caused aristocratic infertility and sickness that began in the Roman Empire around the inception of our period, had already clearly affected the Greeks for several centuries, and must have spread to Asia Minor and Egypt, or to whatever country had a common culture with Rome. The genocultural sterilization was cumulative, reduc-

147

ing the numbers of descendants of the upper class from one
generation to the next, and lowering the genetic level of all
classes, but especially of the richest.

We have already described how the Roman upper classes were continually decimated by lead poisoning, and probably sterilized by overheating of the male genitals, and by
various other factors. A cyclic process of aristothanasia was
drastically depleting the ranks of the genetically and culturally best. The vacancies were filled by upwardly moving
elements, who rose either by ability from the lower classes,
or who were drawn into Rome and the other capitals by the
lure of wealth and power. Each replacement would in turn
be decimated and replaced by new cohorts of the ablest substitutes from below. The Roman supply of talent was continuously being drained, generation after generation for seven
centuries.

Higher Education

The positive association between innate ability on the
one hand and wealth and culture on the other, must have
been unusually high in the Roman Republic and Empire.
The reason was that Rome during this era carried out the
modern democratic ideal of *social mobility* to a higher degree
than in any society known to us, unless it were Greece,
especially Athens, which was already ruined, apparently by
the same process a few centuries earlier. When the growth of
empire, egalitarian attitudes, and the military and civil bureaucracy coincided with a continual dying out of the elite,
there necessarily occurred a great potential for upward mobility among people of talent, men or women. But each promoted generation was in turn ruined by lead.

Sterilization or death, then replacements from below,
to be in turn decimated, involved not only rapid genetic deterioration, but also debasement of culture. For to acquire
higher education and culture usually required two things
simultaneously: youth and money. The upward-moving replacements from the lower classes could rarely acquire that
higher culture which was the birthright of the ancient

aristocracy.

To be sure, higher education in the Roman world was not *quite* the exclusive prerogative of the upper classes. The institutions of higher education corresponding to our universities were to be found in most great cities of the Empire. Their teachers were paid privately, and the best commanded very high fees. Thus Cicero paid 40,000 sesterces a year to send his sons to the university of Athens, which claimed the highest standing for philosophy. One would go to Rhodes for rhetoric, or to Alexandria for medicine. Such higher education was generally beyond the reach of the middle, not to mention the lower classes.

Some private endowments for secondary and higher education did exist, such as one endowed by our Pliny* at Comum, modern Como.[1] And endowed or not (usually not), there were secondary schools teaching chiefly rhetoric and Greek. Trajan provided scholarships for 5,000 poor but talented boys. Under Hadrian, financing of higher education by the cities had become common, as had pension funds for retired teachers. Hadrian and Antoninus exempted the leading professors of the city from taxation.[1] These public subsidies for higher education made it more widely available, but certainly not so much for the poor as today, when free schools are everywhere, even to the university level.

And today cheap reading matter, printed on paper, can be picked up as trash, or borrowed from countless free libraries. Very different from the days when all reading matter had to be written by hand on papyrus, or scratched on tablets.

Incidentally, Roman higher education was available to women, even wives, a privilege that would not reach Germany until the mid-nineteenth century. All in all, we conclude that there were some opportunities for an upwardly mobile commoner to provide higher culture for his children. But how many children would he have who survived? And would he acquire culture himself to match his new status? Not likely.

Immigrants

Still, we cannot claim a progressive decline in the culture of the Roman Empire from 150 B.C. to the fifth century A.D. For countervailing forces were operative. One of these was a partial breakdown of class and national barriers to education and promotion. Another factor was an increase in the demand for highly specialized intellectual activity, both to administer the Empire and to provide cultural facilities for its upper class. This requirement caused a significant expansion in higher education and professional schooling. Both as voluntary immigrants and as slaves, Greek-speaking and to a lesser extent Syrian and Jewish professionals, came to the West, to serve as architects, physicians, writers, artists, and educators. Other men of outstanding ability were attracted to Rome in the hope of rising to fill responsible posts in the management of the Empire. The Asian and African provinces suffered a significant brain drain. To come to Rome, even as a slave, could be a privilege for the skilled, intelligent, and capable. Slaves of this sort found it easy to win their freedom after some years, and they or their descendants might amass wealth, wield political and economic power, and amalgamate with the aristocracy, which was ever dying out and being replaced.

But since the immigrants were as susceptible to sterilization, sickness or death, from lead poisoning, as the Roman intellectuals and administrators whom they replaced, their influx served merely as a palliative, not as a cure. Their presence delayed but could not avert the decay of Roman culture.

Decline of Greece

The Greek and Greek-speaking men of ability who provided Rome with much of her science, and manned most of her professions, came mostly from Asia Minor and Alexandria. In his monumental history of science, Professor George Sarton devotes half a page or more to each of 53 Greek speakers, who made important contributions during the period considered, and to 38 Italians and people of Italian descent. Of the 43 Greeks whose birthplace or residence is listed, 20 came from Asia Minor, 14 from Alexandria, 4 from Greece and Macedonia, 3 from Italy, and 2 from Byzantium.[2] The locus of Greek intellect had decisively shifted from Hellas to the wider domains of the Seleucids and Ptolemies.

Since lead poisoning had already been sterilizing the Greek intellect for several centuries (but likely not so badly in the outlying Hellenized regions) it is not surprising that the greatest achievements of Greek and Hellenistic science antedate our period. Pythagoras, Euclid, Archimedes, and Eratosthenes, the native Greek giants of pre-Renascence mathematics and astronomy, were already past.

The persistence of Greek-writing genius in Alexandria and Asia Minor, despite centuries of exposure to lead poisoning, may have been due to differences in drinking and eating habits. Beer more than wine was the national drink of Egypt. It was second only to vegetable oil as a liquid for consumption. We know that under the Ptolemies the guild of professional brewers was licensed and controlled by the state.[3] While viniculture had long been known in Egypt,[4] an extensive beer-drinking preference may have limited the scope and severity of lead poisoning. Consumption of date wine and similar beverages in Asia Minor and Egypt might also have reduced exposure to lead poisoning.[5]

In Alexandria, however, the Greek population appears to have declined significantly, by one-half according to the third-century bishop and saint Dionysius.[6] If Jews constituted two-fifths of the population of Alexandria by the first century A.D.,[7] the main reason may have been that they were little exposed to sterility by lead poisoning, for they followed the numerous biblical exhortations against heavy drinking.[8] The Jews have always been a sober people; in America their alcoholic rate is one-half of one percent versus eight percent among non-Jews.

Despite a great decline in the population of Greece proper, Greek speakers were able to provide Rome with the great majority of her physical scientists and professionals, until about A.D. 200. The Greek contribution thereafter was primarily in the fields of theology, history, and medicine. Even in these areas there remained few first class minds, and nothing comparable to those who contributed to the explosion of Hellenistic science in the third century B.C.

Sorokin's Measurements of Greco-Roman Creativity

Our conclusions have been corroborated by P. A. Sorokin's analysis of classical creativity, a most important attempt to measure the rates of innovative intellectual activity from earliest times to the beginning of the present century.[9] Sorokin's principal source was Ludwig Darmstaedter's *Handbuch zur Geschichte der Naturwissenschaften und der Technik*, a monumental cooperative endeavor by 26 German specialists, published in 1908. The compilation includes "not only the pioneering creations and fundamental achievements, but also the separate individual steps necessary for a successful production." All the major developments in technology are encompassed. For medicine, Sorokin used as a supplement the more detailed material in F. H. Garrison's *Introduction to the History of Medicine* (1929). Sorokin's compilation deals with discoveries rather than individual scientists. Hence, the simultaneous independent discovery of the same phenomenon has two entries, while a discovery resulting from the cooperative work of more than one thinker is reported as a single event.

For the years 500 B.C. to A.D. 600, Sorokin and Darmstaedter listed 250 major discoveries in science, 101 in technology, and 7 in geographical discovery. Of the scientific achievements, 27 were in mathematics, 47 in astronomy, 37 in biology, 66 in medical science, 20 in chemistry, 51 in physics, and 2 in geology. The most productive century in science, according to these data, was the fourth B.C., after which came a gradual decline, then a secondary peak in the first century A.D. But by A.D. 200 scientific creativity was apparently exhausted. The curve of technology was roughly similar, but reached its all-time peak not in Greek or Hellenistic times but in the Augustan era. The broad course of this ebb and flow of creativity is shown in Table 3 on the next page. For further details, the reader should consult Sorokin's more comprehensive presentation.

Roman Attitudes toward Science and Invention

The traditional Roman attitude toward science and

TABLE 3
GRECO-ROMAN DISCOVERIES
IN SCIENCE, TECHNOLOGY AND EXPLORATION [9]

Period	Discoveries in: Science	Technology	All Discoveries
400-301 B.C.	46	12	60
300-201 B.C.	33	12	45
200-101 B.C.	14	2	17
100-1 B.C.	14	17	32
1- -100 A.D.	39	21	61
101-200 A.D.	23	4	27
201-300 A.D.	5	3	8
301-400 A.D.	8	8	16
401-500 A.D.	2	2	4
Totals	184	81	270

9.   P. A. Sorokin: *Social and Cultural Dynamics,* (Amer. Book Co.),
vol. II, pp. 132-4. The total given, All Discoveries, is a little greater than those of Science plus Technology, because it also includes
a few geographic discoveries.

invention was negative. Following Aristotle, Seneca made a
sharp line of demarcation between the base and the liberal
arts. The former were concerned with the sordid business of
helping man earn a livelihood. The latter were concerned
with "virtue." They were "liberal" because they alone were
worthy of the attention of free men or, as Pliny thot, because
they derived their name from "liberty, the supreme good."[10]
Cicero held similar opinions. He thot workshops and facto-
ries vulgar, trade dishonorable, finance and moneylending
"sordid." Architecture and medicine were somewhat more
honorable, but there was "nothing better, nothing more attractive, nothing more suitable" for a gentleman than farm-
ing.[11]

The traditional Roman attitude toward invention was
almost one of suspicion, or contempt, except in certain un-

commercial, "noble" fields; namely, military and civil engineering, the fine arts, especially architecture, and agriculture, with its related industries. The Roman indifference or even contempt for industrial invention is illustrated by the story of the unfortunate inventor of "an unbreakable type of glass," who demonstrated his discovery to the emperor Tiberius in the hope of a munificent reward. After receiving assurances that nobody else knew of this invention, Tiberius ordered the man's head cut off, on the theory that his improved glass, if put on the market, would cause a catastrophic fall in the price of metals and thus precipitate an economic crisis.[12] The story is told by Petronius, repeated by Pliny,* and garbled by Dio Cassius.[13]

Not all Roman rulers were so shortsighted and averse to change as the "man of resentment," Tiberius. Nero, who had been so much maligned by the patricians and Christians whom he persecuted, had the un-Roman ambition of becoming a great actor and musician; he surrounded himself with artists and intellectuals, was receptive to new ideas, and commenced construction of the Corinth canal. His Golden House was replete with such miraculous technological gadgets as dining rooms "whose panels could turn and shower down flowers," and a main circular banquet hall that "constantly revolved day or night like the heavens."[14]

This tantalizingly incomplete description suggests that Nero was wasting invention in the same way as that great first-century B.C. mathematician and technologist, Heron of Alexandria,[15] who reported, among other things, how to use steam power to make a mechanical bird sing, blow a trumpet, and keep a ball continuously in the air. Heron, who lived in the first century B.C., was probably an Egyptian rather than a Greek. He invented or reported on three forms of heat en-

---

12. While we may question the word of the inventor or of Petronius, the story illustrates a great hindrance to ancient Greco-Roman technology, that its improvement was left to the artisan class, not to those with brains, learning and financial and political power—except in the fields of civil and military engineering, architecture, and agriculture with viniculture and such related industries. Cf. Gilfillan: *Supplement to the Sociology of Invention*, on Why the Classical Age was Uninventive; pp. 163-71, San Francisco Press, 1971.

gine, a water organ, and a slot machine, among others but they were hardly of practical utility. Such inventions were functionally like those of the showman or the chef, who devised new delights for the rich, not helps for industry. So such inventions remained useless and forgotten, instead of revolutionizing industry or transportation. The utterly stupid ancient horse harness, which yoked pairs of horses in such a way that it choked them if they pulled hard, remained practically unchanged for 4,000 years.[16] The most amazingly complicated machine known from antiquity, the Greek mechanical geared calendar of the planets, constructed in 87 B.C. and recovered from the sea off Antikythera, served astronomical and astrological purposes, but had no other use.[17]

Mathematics and the Physical Sciences

Let us begin with the exact sciences, an area in which comparisons can be more objective than in such fields as philosophy, literature, or art.

Consider mathematics and astronomy. The Romans never produced a single figure of importance in either field, until the time of the Egyptian Heron. After him came the towering figure of the Alexandrian Ptolemy, roughly contemporaneous with Marcus Aurelius. During the next century nobody first-rate appeared. Then there came a last flurry, an Indian summer of creativity in the third century A.D. Pappos, an Alexandrian Greek who flourished under Diocletian, systematized and extended Euclidean geometry. His contemporary Diophantos, another Alexandrian Greek, created the system of equations that bears his name; he ranks among the greatest algebraists of all time.

"After the death of Pappos, Greek and indeed all European mathematics lay dormant for about a thousand years,"

---

16. The one exception to that horse harness was that of the Roman *cisium*, far better, like the modern breast harness. Yet for some reason it was never used save for a one-horse cab. Information on the ancient harness is supplied by its "discoverer," R. Lefebvre des Noëttes: *La Force motrice animale à travers les âges,* 1924, and his later studies.

wrote H. W. Turnbull in *The Great Mathematicians*.[18] For ten centuries, there was nobody but two Indian algebraists.[19]

In applied physics and engineering, the Romans played a leading role. While they never learned to equal Indian steel, and were unable to produce silk during the lifetime of the Empire of the West, they led the world in glass manufacture, and in the application of waterpower. They were outstanding in such military engineering specialities as fortifications and siege warfare.[20]

The greatest achievements of Roman engineering date from the earlier centuries, before much lead poisoning had sapped intelligence. The first Roman aqueduct, the Appian, built in 312 B.C., led water partly underground into the Eternal City. The Aqua Marcia (144 B.C.) carried water for six miles, partly on those striking arches Roman engineers had practiced for centuries, in order to keep the water from descending and thus coming under pressure. But when the water *had* to descend—to cross a deep valley or to serve city streets, lead was used wholesale to contain pressure. The 1,300 miles of aqueducts thus created provided Rome with 800,000,000 liters of water daily. Pliny thot these aqueducts Rome's supreme achievement. "Who will venture to compare these mighty conduits with the idle Pyramids or the famous, but useless, works of the Greeks?" Frontinus asked rhetorically.[21] The construction of about 80,000 km of the most durable roads in history was another fantastic achievement of Roman engineering, whose excessive expense was called for by their inefficient horse harness and absence of horseshoes.

Architecture (to be discussed later) and civil engineering reached their peaks in the age of Augustus. Vitruvius who lived then, left ten books of architecture which survive and constitute an encyclopedia of technical knowledge of his day.

---

19. The Arabs did not invent the misnamed Arabic number system, but borrowed it from India. They compiled and translated the work of others, but "lacked the originality and genius of Greece or India." The long slumber of the Western scientific mind began to end only with Leonard of Pisa (1170-1230), who fostered the Arabic system and discovered the Fibonacci series. (Quotation from Turnbull in James R. Newman, ed.: *The World of Mathematics*, Simon & Schuster, 1956, vol. I, p. 118.)

Among other things, he explained that vibrations of the air cause sound. In addition to his work in architectural acoustics, Vitruvius also warned of the danger of lead poisoning from the water supply (see Chapter 6).

Frontinus (A.D.49-103) was superintendent of Rome's water supply, and wrote a definitive work on the system, as well as a basic volume of Roman engineering. One of his discoveries was that impurities in drinking water can be filtered out thru sand.

The last great figure in Roman engineering was Apollodoros of Damascus, a Levantine Greek. He bridged the Danube near the Iron Gate, built Trajan's forum and aqueduct, wrote a book (now lost) on siege warfare, and was judicially murdered by Hadrian. After him there were no more giants in classical engineering.

Polygraphs

From Aristotle onward the classical work was richly endowed with polygraphs, men who wrote on every possible topic, attempting encyclopedias of knowledge. We can hardly place these men in specific sciences, nor evaluate their work, because it is difficult to distinguish original thot from reporting.

The central figure among these polygraphs is Pliny* the Elder (A.D. 23-79), whose immense *Natural History*, an encyclopedia of mixed knowledge and nonsense, we have so often utilized. Varro (116-27 B.C.)[22] wrote books on geometry, arithmetic, grammar, dialectics, astrology, music, medicine, and agriculture. Only those on early Latin and on agriculture (including viniculture) survive. Deemed by Quintillian "the most learned of the Romans," Varro had intimations of the germ theory of disease. He warned people who lived near swamps to take precautions against "certain minute creatures that cannot be seen by the eyes, which float thru the air and

---

22. But he says almost nothing about viniculture, only how vat wine was made, without indication of leading (save from the winepress). I:54.

enter the body thru the mouth and the nose and there cause serious disease." After Varro and Pliny, the classical world boasted few polygraphs.

Medical Writers

After 150 B.C. Greek physicians from Athens, Alexandria, and Asia Minor began to flock to Rome and to dominate the profession. The most prominent figure in the first century A.D. was Celsus, a Roman encyclopedist whose works on philosophy, law, military science, and agriculture are lost. He accurately described the human skeleton, and gave classic accounts of such operations as tonsillectomy and cataract removal. Sarton considers Celsus' work on medicine "a masterly compilation," and after Hippocrates and Galen, ranks Celsus as "the greatest medical work of antiquity."[23]

After Celsus, there are such significant figures in classical medicine as Dioscorides,* a Greek from Tarsus, whose work on pharmacology and medical botany was to dominate those fields for almost fifteen centuries; Rufus of Ephesus, who wrote an important book on the pulse; and Soranus, likewise of Ephesus, who pioneered in gynecology and contraception. Both Rufus and Soranus practiced medicine in Rome.

The last major medical figure, and one of the greatest of Greco-Roman civilization, was Galen (A.D. 129-199), a Greek anatomist, physician, and philosopher from Pergamum. Galen systematized Greek medical thot, and did experimental work to determine the function of kidneys, lungs and cerebrum, and to establish that the arteries carry out the blood. "After Galen's death," writes a modern authority, "the creative process of discussion and dissection tapered off into treatises which took Galen at his word."[24]

Thus, after about 200 A.D., there were no more originative figures in Roman medicine. Instead stood people like Oribasius (ca. 325-400), physician to Julian the Apostate who wrote a seventy-book medical encyclopedia, almost all borrowed from Galen. In medicine as elsewhere in science, decline began early and had almost reached bottom by the third century.[25]

Roman Law

Perhaps the most famous of Rome's legacies to western civilization has been Law. The development of Roman law spanned almost a millenium, from the Twelve Tables of 451 B.C. to the codification of Justinian's *Digest* or *Pandects* in A.D. 533. The European rediscovery of the Justinian codes in the fifteenth century had a profound impact on the development of dynastic power, modern nationalism, and those juridical concepts which western civilization holds in common.

Probably the first of the really great Roman jurists were Publius Mucius Scaevola, who became consul in 133 B.C., and his son, consul in 95 B.C. The Scaevolae were among the first to attempt to organize the vast, unwieldy corpus of Roman edicts, traditional law, and case law, into a coherent unity.

The need for a uniform, comprehensive, internally consistent, logical, and teachable system of law increased as Rome emerged as a great imperial power, administering justice and order to polyglot peoples with differing traditions of local law. Hence the great age of Roman jurists spans the era of imperial consolidation and incipient internal disintegration, stretching from the time of Longinus, roughly a contemporary of Augustus, to the death of Ulpian in A.D. 228.

Thus the age of creativity in Roman law extended about a century after that of the sciences; yet it showed a like decay. By the end of inglorious Caracalla's reign the lights of legal creativity were fading. Half a century later, they were extinguished.

This analysis may seem contradicted by the fact that Justinian's Digest and Code, often regarded as the supreme

25.   In a recent book on Roman medicine, Scarborough: *Roman Medicine,* Cornell Univ. Press, 1969, lists about twice as many Greek as Roman figures in his biographical sketches (pp. 149-61). Of those to whom dates can be assigned, 24 flourished before 150 B.C., 20 between that date and the year 1, 15 in the first century, as many in the 2nd, and only 5 thereafter.

achievement of Roman law, appeared in the first half of the sixth century. But they are merely the final form in which Roman law was digested and presented. They are devoid of originality, for Justinian and his advisors "gloried in the unquestionable absence of all innovation," in everything they did. In fact, in Procopius' *Secret History*, the most serious charge he could make against the emperor he ostensibly served, but privately hated, was that of innovation.[26]

The 2,200 closely printed pages of the German edition of Justinian's *Corpus Juris Civilis* contain 9,142 citations and excerpts from previous authorities. While some of those writers may have been mere popularizers and compilers, the weight they receive in the *Corpus* may be indicative of their importance as legal thinkers.

Ulpian (Domitius Ulpianus of Syria), whose greatest claim to fame is not his original contributions but his ability as a compiler and encyclopedist of the law, stands in first place, with 2,464 extracts. His career was cut short when he was murdered by his praetorians in A.D. 228.

Second place goes to Julius Paulus, probably a contemporary of Ulpian, with 2,081 citations. He was a Praetorian Prefect and perhaps more a philosopher of the law than a legal analyst. About a sixth of Justinian's *Digest* derives from him. The third most cited legal mind is that of AEmilius Papinianus, also a high official, whose legal work is noted for its precision and close reasoning. Papinianus has 601 citations. He was murdered by order of emperor Caracalla for refusing to condone one of the assassinations perpetrated by that tyrant.

Pomponius, who died in 138, stands in fourth place, with 578 citations. Finally, with 535 references, there is Gaius, about whom almost nothing is known. It was said he wrote "a lucid, elementary handbook that found favor," and was widely disseminated. F. A. Hayek then concluded "When the later men became incapable of handling the great treatises, elementary books grew in importance, and this book, with others of the same type, mostly abridged, sufficed for them."[27]

Thus, in law as elsewhere, there is overwhelming evidence that a collapse of creativity occurred at least by the opening decades of the third century, and likely earlier.

Historians

Rome's pride in her imperial achievements inspired historians and biographers, from Ennius in the second century B.C. to Procopius seven centuries later. But as always the record shows an ultimate decline of genius. The consensus of modern historians is that Tacitus (55-120 A.D.) stands head and shoulders above all other classical historians since Thucydides. His only possible rivals are Polybius (207-145 B.C.), Josephus (A.D. 37-100), Suetonius (ca. A.D. 75-160), who was more an assembler of gossip and anecdotes than a serious-minded biographer, and Dio Cassius (ca. A.D. 155-240). But after him we have mostly lackluster church historians, whose tendentious studies are enlivened by numerous accounts of supernatural occurrences. Finally, there came Procopius, who secretely believed that his master, the Emperor Justinian, was either the anti-Christ, or at the very least, "a demon in human form."[28]

Literature

The old Republican days of Rome had produced some very solid writers. The dramatists Plautus (d. 184 B.C.), Ennius (d. 169 B.C.) and the serious historian and statesman Cato (d. 149 B.C.) whose works on viniculture we have consulted; Terence (d. 159 B.C.), a dramatist of Carthaginian slave origin; Cicero (d. 45 B.C.) for his fine orations and other prose; Caesar, for his famous history of the conquest of Gaul; and the philosopher Lucretius (d. 55 B.C.).

The greatest period of Roman literature was the Golden Augustan Age (42 B.C.-A.D. 17), with its immortally shining lights, the poets Vergil and Horace and the historian Livy. The period dubbed the Silver Age (to A.D. 130) was an era still able tho not so brilliant, its stars the martyred philosopher Seneca, his son of the same name, the historian Tacitus, and Pliny* the Elder, whose credulous but prodigiously

encyclopedic *Natural History*, finished in 77 A.D., we have
so often used.

The insane, probably lead-poisoned emperor Nero
was both a patron of culture, and a ruler who shortened the
life-span of many men of letters. He put Lucan to death for
conspiracy, killed the enlightened and humane essayist Seneca (A.D. 65), and probably also dispatched Petronius, ending
the career of a supreme satirist whose *Satyricon* can be considered an embryonic form of the novel.

The earlier Antonines boasted such figures as the
rhetorician Pliny the Younger (ca. 62-113), the priggish and
affected nephew of our encyclopedist. Epictetus (60-120), a
largely self-educated Greek slave and Stoic philosopher, was
an enlightened opponent of some of Rome's most respected,
inhuman, institutions. The literary tone of the age was set by
the savage and defeatist satires of Martial (42-102) and Juvenal (60-140). The latter is said to have condemned every established Roman institution except gladiators.

The decline in literature became precipitous under
the later Antonine emperors. But the *Meditations* of the
great emperor Marcus Aurelius (121-180) are an exception to
this generalization, as are the tales of Apuleius. A more re-
presentative figure is Aulus Gellius (117-180), who combined
a love of archaic language with an absorbing interest in trivia.

After Hadrian's reign came only writers characterized
by a superficial and mediocre style, all too often filled with
tortuous, empty rhetorical embellishment, a style that would
become *de riguer* in formal Byzantine writing. Fronto (ca.
100-170), an African, wrote forensic speeches, and tracts on
such topics as "Praises of Smoke and Dust." Aulus Gellius
(ca. 130-180) was the prototype of Byzantine compilers and
encyclopedists, amassing piles of information with not the
slightest conception of order nor of clarity in style and
composition.

For in the eastern, Greek-writing half of the Empire,
the decadence was parallel. Even as early as the first century
A.D. the only examples of scholarship worthy of the name
are the neoPlatonic mystical tracts of Philo of Alexandria. In
the period from Nerva to Trajan, there was a brief revival in

the *genre* of the novel; yet these works (by Heliodorus, Achilles Tatius, or Longus) are all characterized by an artificial insipid, and diffuse style.

Other branches of literature were effectively dead by the end of the second century: the theater was extinct, its function having been absorbed by the spectacles of the mystery cults, suggestive of later liturgies. Poetry waned into insignificance. The historians of the period, like Appian, Dio Cassius, Herodian, and Dexippus, all focussed on the history of Rome, yet their works were conceived and executed with a mediocrity that allows no comparison to masters like Thucydides, Tacitus or Polybius. In the Greek East, the sole areas of literary creativity seem to have been limited to the moralists like Plutarch and Lucian, and the philosophers Plotinus (d. 270) and Porphyry. NeoPlatonism was a philosophy of mysticism, inner-worldliness, and alienation from this world— a far cry from the confidence of classical philosophy.

The development of Latin literature, after the third century—from Constantine and into the fifth century—shows some minor signs of revival, but the impoverishment of the previous centuries had left an irreversible impact. In traditional *genres* like the panegyric (e.g., Eumenas), or imperial biography (e.g., Spartianus, Vulcacius, Gallicanus), the baroque inflation of the past continued. In content, they reflect little concern for an accurate representation of their objects of praise or study. To the historian, they are useless. In history, Ammianus Marcellinus (d. 400) represents the last pagan historian of antiquity. Ammianus himself had an impartial and inquiring mind, and was an eye-witness of much he wrote about. Yet his style is laborious and convoluted, and his "history" filled with a plethora of imaginary speeches in flamboyant rhetoric.

In other *genres*, like poetry and epistolography, a few names stand out like isolated lamps alight in the night. Ausonius (d. 395) and Claudian (d. 408) wrote poems of minor merit; Claudian was noted for his sycophancy, declamations, and invectives against enemies of his patrons. The themes of the poetry of dying antiquity had none of the vigor and loftiness that inspired Vergil. Thus the period of literary history we have surveyed represents continuing atrophy.

The Visual Arts

In Architecture and the other visual arts cultural decline was perhaps slower, and certainly less evident than in
fields that required more individuality and innovation. Pro-
ceeding within the limitations of a rigorous tradition, the
architects of the Antonine era were able to create numerous
great, somewhat novel, and beautiful structures. The vast
Greco-Roman City of the Sun at Baalbek in Lebanon, probably not completed until the third century, rivaled in splen-
dor and beauty any edifice the Romans ever built, but dis-
played no innovation, save in size.[29]

Most inventive was the noble Pantheon (Plate 20 on
page 80), rebuilt under Hadrian in 110-125. Its great masonry dome 43.5 in. in diameter, was open at the center, and
rested on a cylindrical wall topped by a covered iron chain
(instead of buttresses) to counter the radial outward thrust,
probably the first example of reinforced concrete. This religious structure is in use to this day. Later architecture showed
no novelties during the epoch considered.

In sculpture, the technical ability of earlier ages was
not lost until after the age of the Antonines. The portrait
heads of Nerva and of Antinous, which his homosexual lover,
the emperor Hadrian commissioned, rival the sculpture of
more creative ages. After the Antonines however, from about
A.D. 180 on, the tendency was for Roman sculpture to
become lifeless, wooden, and lacking in individualization.

But there is the Arch of Constantine, you may say; a
great work of art, of a rather late date—312 A.D. Yes, great,
an arch—something-or-other, so we have illustrated it in Plate
17 on page 77. Now let us consider it closely. Its design, an
arch of triumph, was old; there were several in Rome, including the *triple* arch of Septimius Severus. The fine sculptures
with which Constantine's structure is adorned had been *torn
bodily* from earlier monuments of Trajan, Hadrian, Marcus
Aurelius, and other previous emperors. And where the booty
included a portrait of an emperor, his face was rechiseled to

look like Constantine's, who was beardless. A good job for a stonemason, to play barber to a bearded emperor.

The one sculpture on the arch that is original is a long, narrow band showing Constantine addressing his Senate. The senators are shown from their backs, and each man is depicted identically, each like two gobs of mud, a round gob for the head, resting on a broader gob for the shoulders. To be sure, the arch was built hurriedly; but there was no necessity for haste in erecting this supreme tribute to the emperor and his empire.

What does such "art" tell us about the culture and brains of the authorities who ordered it and the "artists" who designed it? Does not this great, supreme arch, when looked at closely, become a monument to pitiful decadence? Some wealth still remains, and some memories of "the glory that was Greece, and the grandeur that was Rome," but no more capacity to create, but only to copy or to steal, from the monuments of their past which was past.

It is harder to tell the story of ancient *painting*, since it has hardly survived save at Pompeii and Herculaneum. (See Plates 18 and 19 on pages 78-79.) But we may infer that that disaster of A.D. 79 was about at the artistic peak. Some 3,500 frescoes have been found in Pompeii. more than survive from all the rest of the Greco-Roman world. Altho Pompeii was a rather unimportant city, one may assume that its artists represent nearly the best of Roman painting. They testify to the vigor, realism, and genius of ordinary artists of the Augustan Age, and of the era of the Claudian and Flavian rulers during the remaining years of the first century.

After about 100 A.D. we witness a failure of creativity in Roman painting, similar to what we have encountered in other fields. Of course there are exceptions to the general decline, such as the realistic portraiture of the Fayyûm, possibly the work of beer-drinking Egyptian artists whose ancestry had not suffered so much from lead.

Gladiators

This pecularly Roman institution (tho learned from

the Etruscans) began early, at least by 264 B.C., but developed most in the much later period of intellectual decadence. Then the gladiatorial spectacles invaded not only all the public arenas, like the Colosseum, but also extended even to private entertainments, with as many as a hundred pairs of gladiators fighting. The emperor Claudius was devoted to the arena, and Nero and Titus put on prodigious shows. Under Nero even Senators and well-born women occasionally appeared as gladiators, and sometimes emperors entered the arena, tho doubtless with precautions against being the victim. Gladiators often served in bands as protectors for noblemen in the Roman streets. They were well fed, so presumably well leaded.

All this love of violence, evidenced probably also in the civil wars, could come from our old saturnine poison, lead. For two of its symptoms are hyperactivity and violence (see Chapter 7). Christianity finally ended gladiatorial combats.

Drinking Contests

The last evidence of upper class decadence, of which we shall write, was the introduction of drinking contests, followed by self-induced vomiting, after which one could proceed to eat and drink more. Of course such activities were not for the poor. The "king of the feast" might prescribe ten cups of wine to be drunk by each man present. (To be sure, the wine was always diluted, in what proportion the "king" would prescribe.) Again, a man might take a challenge to drink as many cups of wine as were called for by a throw of the dice. And there were contests as to who could drink the most.

Some would take emetics to induce vomiting, a custom G. H. Ellwanger says came from Egypt.[30] And occasionally, Pliny says, a man would first drink hemlock in order to drive himself to swill greater draughts of wine, for fear of death.[31]

Such customs appear to have arisen around the first century A.D. Horace does not mention them. Surely not many ideas are stupider than to fill oneself with wine, water, and food in order to vomit them up and then repeat this all over again. It was during the reign of Tiberius (A.D. 14-37) that the fashion of drinking on an empty stomach began. Claudius (41-54) and Vitellius (69) were the only emperors we find mentioned as habitually using emetics.

This behavior has a double connection with lead. For crazy ideas, as well as nausea and vomiting after eating or drinking, are signs of lead poisoning.[32]

So much eating and drinking among the rich might lead us to expect them to be fat. Yet we rarely read of overweight people, or see them in ancient sculptures or paintings. The explanation could be that one of the signs of lead poisoning is fat's opposite, emaciation.

Summary of the Creative Decline

In *philosophy*, the Romans were imitators and interpreters. By 150 B.C. the great age of Greek philosophy had come to an end. The only major subsequent figure was Plotinus (203-270), the Egyptian NeoPlatonist.

In *social organization* the most marked change came in the late third century: Diocletian's useless bureaucratic rigidities, one of which required every man to follow the occupation of his father. The "free" population was divided into two castes, the *honestiores* and the *humiliores*. The latter were treated almost like slaves, and might be beaten or sometimes branded. There were ever heavier taxes, maintaining a lavish court and a near worship of the emperor, which did indeed make civil wars less frequent.[33]

To sum up, the creative processes that advance culture reached an apparent peak in the Augustan Age, underwent a slow decline in the first century of the Christian era, fell faster during the second century, were largely exhausted by A.D. 200, and sank ever lower for centuries thereafter. The movement of decay varied in timing and rapidity from one field to another, but the general rule was that the more intellectually exacting the creative area, the swifter the degeneration and the more total the collapse.

The causative agency with which we are concerned was chiefly lead poisoning, which had begun centuries earlier among the Greek and Hellenized peoples of the Mediterranean, but which likely hit the Romans especially around the middle of the second century B.C. The cultural decay of the classical world was wrot by lead and some other factors, which reduced the numbers of people capable of specialized higher learning, so necessary to run, improve, educate and entertain the great empire. The great brains were searched for everywhere. Able and educated men flocked to Rome, or were imported as slaves. More and more professions and even the bureaucracy were opened to aliens, freedmen, and slaves. But the people promoted and transplanted to the capitals, to contribute their genius to the Roman system, were themselves exposed to the same sinister, largely saturnine influences. So they left ever fewer descendants to carry on their genes and their culture. The processes of decline worked slowly, and took centuries to accomplish the ruin, but they worked inexorably.

1.   Will Durant: *Caesar and Christ*, 1944, p. 368.
2.   George Sarton: *Introduction to the History of Science*, vol. 1, From Homer to Omar Khayyam, (Wash., Carnegie Inst., 1927).
3.   M. Rostovtzeff: *Social and Economic History of the Hellenistic World*, (Oxford U. Press, 1942), vol. 1, p. 308.
4.   Ibid., vol. 1, pp. 353-355, 1252.
5.   Pliny,* XIV, 19.
6.   Eusebius: *Ecclesiastical History*, VII:21.
7.   Salo Wittmayer Baron: *A Social and Religious History of the Jews*, vol. 1, Ancient Times, Part I, (Columbia U. Press, 1952), pp. 171, 371.
8.   Leviticus X:9; Numbers VI:3; Proverbs XX:1, XXXI:4; Habakuk II:15.
9.   F. A. Sorokin: *Social and Cultural Dynamics*, (Amer. Book Co.), vol. II, pp. 132-4. The total given, All Discoveries, is a little greater than those of Science plus Technology, because it also includes a few geographic discoveries.
10.   Pliny,* XIV, 1, 5.
11.   Quoted by R. H. Barrow: *The Romans*, (Lon., Penguin, 1949), pp. 141-2.

12. See the note on page 154.

13. Petronius: *Satyricon*, chap. 51; Pliny,* XXXVI:26; and Dio Cassius: *History of Rome*, XVII:21.

14. Suetonius: *Lives of the Caesars*, VI. 31.

15. Sarton: op. cit., vol. 1, p. 208.

16. See the note on page 155.

17. Derek de Solla Price: Gears from the Greeks: *Trans. Amer. Philos. Soc.*, n.s. 64, Part 7, 1974; reviewed by A. G. Drachman in *Technology & Culture*, 17:112-6.

18. James R. Newman (ed.): *The World of Mathematics*, Simon & Schuster, 1956, vol. I, p. 117.

19. See the note on page 156.

20; Wm. H. McNeill: *Rise of the West*, Univ. of Chgo. Press, 1963, p. 358.

21. Frontinus: *On the Aqueducts of Rome*, Book I, p. 16.

22. See the note on page 157.

23. Sarton, supra, I:240.

24. Jn. Scarborough: *Roman Medicine*, Cornell U. Press, 1969, p. 51.

25. See the note on page 159.

26. Procopius: *Secret History*, VIII:12, 22-27, and XVIII. Cited in P. N. Ure: *Justinian and his Age*, 1951, pp. 175-7.

27. F. A. Hayek: *Law, Legislation and Liberty*, vol. 1, *Rules* and *Rules and Order*, Univ. of Chgo. Press, 1973, p. 83. Also Theodor Mommsen: *Abriss des römischen Staatsrechts*, 1893, p. 319.

28. Procopius, supra.

29. G. Rodenwaldt: The Transition to Late Classical Art: *Cambridge Ancient History*, 12:551.

30. G. H. Ellwanger: *The Pleasures of the Table*, an account of gastronomy from ancient times, 477 pp., 1902.

31. Pliny,* 14:28.

32. Amer. Pub. Health Asn., Com'ee on Lead: *Occupational Lead Exposure and Lead Poisoning*, 1943, 67 pp., p. 50.

33. V. Gordon Childe: *What Happened in History*, 1942.

13

Lead in Other Countries

Carthage

Carthaginian history (with the Phoenicians, their fore-fathers), are topics which we cannot go into at any length nor conclusively, but in which there are strong indications of dysgenic lead poisoning similar to that in Greece and Rome, plus another and shocking dysgenic factor,[1] the sacrifice of noble children to their gods. Aside from religion, their civilization and technology seem to have been similar to that of their neighbors, the Jews, Syrians, Greeks, Etruscans and Romans. The Romans considered them uncouth. They produced no literature, their art was always poor, they never seemed to excel in anything but trade, navigation, conquest of barbarians, and they produced only one man of genius, Hannibal.

We hear of only one book of theirs, a work on agriculture in 28 "books" by Mago, which the Roman Senate had translated into Latin after the destruction of Carthage. And there was a Greek who translated eight of Mago's "books." Altho these are all lost now, we have found references to Mago's work by four Roman authors. After naming a page-full of Roman writers on agriculture, Varro said Mago surpassed them all, and cited him four times more. Columella* called him the Father of Agriculture, cited him 18 times, and gave his method for making *passum*, raisin wine.[2] A page or two later he indicated leading by some people using old rainwater boiled down, but it is not clear that this Roman practice was also Mago's.

It seems likely that the Carthaginians had the same fatal taste for lead as the Romans. Yet Mago may have had some idea of its harm, since he is cited cooking pomegranates very briefly in seawater, and for his saying that vessels for storing preserves using vinegar or hard brine should be of earthenware or glass.[3] On the whole, we have strong suggestions, tho not proofs, that the Carthaginians mostly shared the Greeks' and Romans' fatal customs in fruit drinks.

But our best evidence for this comes from Clinical Necromancy. Our only bone from Carthage, now Tunisia, is of a rich and leaded person. (See Appendix B on page 192.) And 70 years ago Rosenblatt*[4] found definite lead in his four Carthaginian bones dating from before and after the conquest by Rome.

The horrible Carthaginian custom of sacrificing the eldest sons of noble families, by strangling and then burning them to satisfy the gods Melkart-Moloch, or Tanit, has been discussed by our distinguished eugenic scholar Weyl.[1] While some historians used to consider it largely a calumny by the Romans, the statements of Diodorus of Sicily (ca. 20 B.C.) have been verified by the 1963 discovery, in a Punic (Carthagian) cemetery on Sardinia, of the bones of 3000 children from one month to four years old, with inscriptions stating that they were the first-born sons of noble families. Likewise the bones of thousands of very young children have been found at Carthage. If from that city 500 boys from the top five percent of the population were sacrificed every five years, Weyl guesses that this would have exterminated one-fifth of the wealthy from each generation. Along with the high death rates of ancient times, especially among lead-affected children and their rich parents, this child sacrifice would have been a very serious additional factor for aristocide.

Normally there would be a *eugenic* force in all countries, in that the upper class tend to have more sons than daughters, as we explained in Chapters 10 and 11, and men can have more children than women can. Other eugenic factors are that high-ranking men tend to have first choice of females, and would tend to have more mates and offspring than the poorer males, both by births and by easier survival. But these factors were partly blocked and reversed in Carthage, by burning up for Melkart so many sons of the nobility.

Greece

About the same race-molding factors seem to have ruled and ruined Greece as at Rome, from lead used in the same baleful ways by the upper class (except for lead-glazed pottery, which they received after the disappearance of their genius). They had hot bathing as well, but not a dangerous change of men's costume. Yet we have not meant to positively claim, nor attempted to *prove*, the geno-cultural bane for Greece. Let some other scholar, far more learned than we in that country's history, language and glorious arts, take up this task. It will not be too hard, with so many citations already collected by Hofmann, Rosenblatt, Kobert and Stevenson. He can use clinical necromancy too, especially by finding earlier bones than our single case of a rich person from a tomb of the eighth century B.C., who was but lightly leaded. (See No. 72AA on page 196.) Most of those of the classical and later Greek periods were heavily poisoned.

One source among many that researchers can check is Athenaeus* (I:31) echoing Pliny, and citing Greek wines that produced various symptoms of lead poisoning, including one from Troizene which would make a pregnant woman miscarry, even if she but ate the grapes of that region. Of course, this last assertion was false, but the fanciful exaggeration points to fatally genocidal vintage wine in that region. And in Greece as a whole it looks as if the poor were decimated as well as the rich (tho also from lack of capable people to lead them), because it appears that the whole population of Greece declined to one-tenth. Pausanias' second century A.D. historical guide book to Greece, which is so interesting to us today, mentions no events at all happening in Greece after the Roman conquest of Corinth in 146 B.C.

To be sure, after the sudden death of Greek genius around 320 B.C., Greece occasionally produced useful writers like Plutarch and Polybius, as we have told in Chapter 12. Other good work appeared in the populous eastern regions to which the Greek literary language spread, like the useful but not artistic works of Pausanias, Heron, Athenaeus* and Ptolemy. But these writers can hardly be credited to the Greek *race;* and their ancestors may also have used lead, etc., disastrously.

Persia

Another country of much interest is Persia. When Alexander was living in that empire he conquered, and was becoming alcoholic, insane, violent, and dead at age 33, perhaps he was becoming lead poisoned on Persian or Greek wines.[5]

Egypt

Egypt is a country particularly inviting for study from its relative isolation, and its abundance of documentary and clinical necromantic data on its ruling class, preserved not simply in bones never burnt, but in mummified flesh and blood. In these a high incidence of caries has been noted, a lead symptom. They had wine for the rich, from grapes or dates, and beer for the poor; and they had lead-lined pots, and grape syrup; two jars of it were found in Tut-Ankh-Amen's tomb, and wine that was analyzed. Pliny[6] mentions an Egyptian wine which produced miscarriage. They posessed lead from pre-dynastic times; and they had a kind of lead glaze from 2000 B.C., quite different from the glaze which became popular around 1 A.D. in the Roman Empire. Galena or sometimes lead carbonate made eye paint in Egypt.[7]

What is singularly suggestive about Egypt is that its civilization four times fell back to near barbarism after the V Dynasty (which was the Pyramid age), and also after the XII and the XVIII Dynasties, and in the Ptolemaic age about 200 B.C. Did the saturnine metal weaken their civilization and/or some other factor malefic to geno-culture? Whatever it was should not be too hard for an Egyptologist to find out, especially with hundreds of mummies of the ruling class available for examination, and plenty of physicians who could diagnose not only their likely cause of death, but much of their whole life history, as some have already done.[8]

During Egypt's first debacle, Ipuwer wrote bewailing the civil wars and disorder, the decline of population and the unfruitfulness of women. Schwidetzky[9] has ably considered the genetic history of the Egyptians and many other peoples. Dr. Stevenson's unique *History of Lead Poisoning*[10] gives five pages and thirteen citations to Egypt and Mesopotamia, incidentally citing lead pipes and vases, and up to twenty percent of lead in bronze there. Weyl[11] says skulls of the IV Dynasty averaged 1532 cc. capacity, of the X Dynasty 1400, and in modern Egypt 1348 cc. Our own single bone from Egypt, of a rich person of the Ptolemaic era about 200 B.C., shows hardly any lead. (See Appendix B on page 196.)

Mesopotamia

Another important country of history is Mesopotamia, on which leads to lead can be found in Stevenson*[10] and elsewhere.[12]

Some Modern Lead Researchers

Detlev Stöfen[13] is working on a good idea, that lead poisoning effected not only the earliest civilizations, but also pre-literate barbarism, and even the Stone Age, from the first uses of lead in any form. One early use was likely as a cosmetic. Our modern lead burden has risen to be 100 to 400 times greater than the natural, as Patterson and Salvia[14] have shown. Erich Fromm's *Anatomy of Human Destructiveness*, 1973, provides evidence that the peacefulness of aborigines is higher, the more primitive the tribe. The sadism on New Guinea might be explained by the high geochemical lead in that island.

---

12. V. G. Childe: *New Light on the Most Ancient East*, p. 142, refers to leaden bowls from Jemdet Nasr graves at Ur. And R. C. Thompson refers to red and white lead having been probably used in Assyrian medicine, the latter internally, *On the Chemistry of the Ancient Assyrians*, London, 1925, pp. 88 ff.

1. Weyl: Some Possible Genetic Implications of Carthaginian Child Sacrifice: *Perspectives in Biol. & Med.*, 12:69-78, 1968.
2. Columella,* XII:39 and 42.
3. Ibid., XII:14.
4. Rosenblatt,* pp. 65-70, cases 14-17.
5. J. J. Modi: *Wine among the Ancient Persians*, 16 pp., 1886; in Univ. of Naples library, well worth seeing.
6. Pliny,* XIV:22.
7. Alf. Lucas: *Ancient Egyptian Materials and Industries*, 1926, 1934.
8. Melchiorre Masali, B. Chiarelli & D. Davide: Ricerche sulle collezioni antropologiche egiziane dall'Istituto di Antropologia di Torino; 6 articles in *Rivista di Antropologia*, 1966-8.
   Also Brothwell* and Wells.*
9. Ilse Schwidetzky: Racial Psychology: *Mankind Quarterly*, 2:10-12, 1961; or in her *Menschenbild der Biologie*, 1959, pp. 145-6; or Assortment and Selection: *Social Research*, 1969, Winter, 542-8; or *das Problem des Völkertodes*, 165 pp., Stuttgart, Enka, 1954
10. Stevenson,* Appendix B: Egypt and Mesopotamia, pp. 412-416.
11. Nathaniel Weyl: The Arab World: *Mankind Quarterly*, 8:29.
12. See the note on page 174.
13. Co-author with H. A. Waldron of *Sub-clinical Lead Poisoning,* Academic Press, Lon. & NY, 1974.
14. C. C. Patterson & J. D. Salvia: Lead in the Modern Environment— How much is natural? *Scientist and Citizen*, 10:66-79, 1968.

14

The Fall of Rome

The Fall of Rome, the break-up of the Empire, its conquest by barbarians from the north, is the first thing that comes to peoples' minds when they hear of our discovery. Yet we have never mentioned these matters, unless to specifically exclude them from our theme. But that Fall is probably the most famous event of all history; whole books have been written to explain it, and even the editors of the *Journal of Occupational Medicine*, whose version of our article has been the principal source of all the subsequent immense publicity,[1] entitled it, *"Lead Poisoning and the Fall of Rome."*

To be sure, the declines of genius, progress, prestige, population and potent leadership, which lead poisoning had helped to bring about, were factors in that Fall. But our book must have limits, as our personal capacity has also its bornes, So we shall discuss the other factors in the Fall only in order to mention what they might have been. We shall not try to pronounce on their validities nor weights. But we should point out where some of them had connections with lead poisoning or other factors for genetic and cultural degradation.[2]

2.   The defeat and break-up of the Empire might have been beneficial to mankind, from setting up additional cultures and possible sources of progress. China has at various times been conquered by barbarous peoples, who instead of destroying her culture, adopted and carried it onward. But the degradation of culture which the Roman world underwent before the Fall, and which continued downward after it by lead and other dysgenic factors, were world-hurting harms. If all the other factors for break-up and impoverishment had happened, except the dysgenic, the Empire might have split up into smaller nations, with little or no decline of culture, and more different fields for good innovations to sprout in.

So now let us first merely list those often-discussed probable factors for the Fall, showing some interconnections, and expatiating only on the group which had some relations to lead and other dysgenic factors.

1. *Racial Change.* As the Germani, and the Celts and and Picts in Britain acquired more civilization, military craft, and population, they pressed harder on the Romans. Then as they, as well as the Nordics and the Levantines, entered the Roman military and political service, they doubtless tended to weaken its Roman nationalism.

2. *Climatic Change.* As Ellsworth Huntington proved in one great book after another,[3] the climate of the Mediterranean countries and western Asia has been constantly changing, its spring rainfalls can be measured from year to year by the growth rings of the big trees in California and by other means; and these changes have had wide and profound effects. Above all in west central Asia, loss of summer rainfall caused the pastoral Huns to press upon the Chinese and the Slavs; the latter then pressed on the Germani, who pressed on the Romans. And similarly later with the Arabs upon the Christians. The loss of rain, especially in the summer, not only hurt southern agriculture, but also entailed a loss of the cold fronts, or cyclonic storms as Huntington called them. This seems essential to highest civilization (except along the southern California coast, whose climate is so ideal otherwise). They bring a temporary negative ionization of the air.

Huntington's graphs of the Mediterranean rainfall show a great deterioration from 400 to 210 B.C., partly recouped around 100 B.C., followed by a rather steady decline from 80 A.D. to 450, and remaining low save for brief peaks around 1000 A.D. and 1330.

3. *Soil Exhaustion.* Simkhovich proved great decline in the yield of crops,[4] but it would be hard to separate this factor from the decrease of rainfall.

4. *Deforestation* was another factor, caused partly by climatic change, and partly by men's axes. Wood was a prime necessity, for heat, structure, ships, etc.

5. *Exhaustion of silver*, the only good money, thru wear, loss and trading it to the East for silk, etc., and by the

mines reaching their deepest feasible depth at the time, as
told in our second chapter. At the same time this checked
the far greater flood of lead, since the two metals were mined
together.[5]

6. *Malaria* was a disease of prime importance in the
ancient Mediterranean world, but perhaps more eugenic than
dysgenic. It occurred in swampy, unhealthy country districts
more than cities, and probably affected the poor more than
the rich, especially if the poor wore less clothing and so were
more exposed to mosquito bites. Probably originating in
Africa where the negroes are partly protected from it by sick-
el-cell anemia, it early spread to Asia and to Greece, before
the time of Hippocrates, and thence to Italy. It was especially
bad in the Campanian marshes just south of Rome, and its
incidence in that city has been plotted.[6] It was severe in the
fifth to third centuries B.C., then rose in the fifth to seventh
A.D., and again in the eleventh to thirteenth, and the eighteenth and nineteenth. Climatic and agricultural change were
likely factors. However bad its effects on civilization, Weyl[7]
considers its genetic effect to have been on the whole favor-
able, since the more capable people will quit the region.

Other large parts of the Empire have been free from
malaria, where any one of three requisites; stagnant water,
the anopheles mosquito, or the parasites, were absent.

7. *The Plagues.* The first one, possibly smallpox,
raged between 164 and 189 A.D. and killed our philosopher-
emperor Marcus Aurelius. The Plague of Cyprian was possibly
ergotism from rye, and appeared in 250. Cartwright believes
it "indisputably changed the course of history."[8] The widest
and worst of all the plagues was the bubonic one of the sixth
century, but this came later than the scope of this chapter.

The plagues decreased the military power of the Empire, and the number of its inventors, writers, etc., but need
not have lowered much of its genius, art nor progressiveness,
which we found so markedly decadent. Compare Athens and
Rome at their respective greatest epochs. Rome was far
ahead in population, wealth and other economic parameters,
but Athens was far ahead in genius and its works.

8. We see nothing in Gibbons' suggestion that *Christ-*

ianity helped ruin Rome, but we have told in Chapter 11 the religion's connection with the Levantine population influx.

9. *Cyclic Theories*, such as Spengler's, Gini's, or Toynbee's, regarding nations or cultures changing by a standard process. Such theories are so vague in their definition of what is the nation or culture, and what is its end, that they can prove any case their author takes up. It seems to us that any proved Laws of History must be based on counts and measures of cases happening to defined types of people, such as all people speaking certain mutually comprehensible dialects, or peoples accepting a single authority, or inhabiting a certain unaltered territory. These historians' explanations of particular histories may well be acceptable, but their general laws have never been formulated and established.

Further thots on the proving of Laws of History are expressed in our Appendix D.

10. *Stupid Mistakes of Roman Government*, such as in the last days of the Empire: oppressive taxation, or bureaucratic rigidities like requiring sons to follow the occupation of their fathers, and above all the civil wars of two periods. We discussed these last in our tenth chapter. There we told how the Empire had 420 years of domestic peace, under a Republic guaranteeing preeminence to the patrician *gentes*. It then fell into frequent wars from 87 to 29 B.C. This led to the abandonment of all elections, and finally to sanctification of the imperial throne by Augustus. The second major period of civil wars, from 192 A.D. to the Empire's end in 476, spelled ever-repeated assassinations, civil wars and proscriptions.

Conclusion

We conclude therefore that a marked decline in brain power (which fosters culture) occurred in the Roman ruling classes. This helped to explain the civil wars, the barbarian invasions, and most other losses of a material kind in Roman culture. The direct result of Rome's ruined culture was the disasters of the Dark Ages and the Byzantine stagnation. This result came not so much from the causes enumerated above, but from lead poisoning and other dysgenic factors, which destroyed both the intellect and fertility of the ruling classes who had built the Roman Republic.

1.   See the description of this publicity on page 6.
2.   See the note on page 176.
3.   Ellsworth Huntington: *The Pulse of Asia,* 1907; *Palestine and its Transformation,* 1911; *Civilization and Climate,* 1915-73 eds.; and with S. S. Visher: *Climatic Changes,* 1922.
4.   V. Simkhovich: Hay and History: *Pol. Sci. Qtly.,* 28:3-31, 1913.
5.   C. C. Patterson: Silver Stocks and Losses in Ancient and Medieval Times: *Econ. Hist. Rev.,* 25:205-35, 1972, Table 12. Also from Patterson: Lead in the Environment: in *Lead Poisoning in Man and the Environment,* papers by Eva L. Jernigan et al, NY, Mss. Info. Cp., 1973, pp. 71-87; see 71.
6.   E. H. Ackerknecht: *Short History of Medicine,* tr. 1968, from the German of 1963.
7.   N. Weyl: Disease as a Eugenic Force: *Mankind Qtly.,* 16:243-56 & 304, 1976; 254-6 on malaria.
8.   Fredk. F. Cartwright: *Disease and History.*

Appendices

Appendix A

Explanation of Bone Analyses

Introduction

Prof. Clair C. Patterson, a geochemist at the California Institute of Technology in Pasadena (LCIT in our abbreviations) and the leading analyst of early lead production as well as today's environmental lead, has been engaged to measure for us the lead content of most of our significant bone samples. He has supplied us with more information than we know how to utilize; others, however, might find useful this information transcribed in Appendix B. Professor Patterson's full records may be obtained by serious scientists from the Smithsonian repository, as told in Appendix H. These details include the exact part of the bone that was analyzed by LCIT, the ppm of lead, the percent of lead in the dirt removed from the bone, or in the bone ash or dirt ash, the percentage of copper (Cu) in the bone, and often the percentage of the other poisonous metals, silver (Ag), cadmium (Cd), or zinc (Zn). Prof. Patterson has also been very helpful in advising the author and has written the report that comprises the first part of this Appendix to explain how he coped with the problem of posthumous lead, intrusive from the soil. The methods of the Kettering Laboratory, whose analyses are designated by LKK or LKY, did not distinguish this posthumous leading from that ingested during life.

Effects of Lead from the Soil on Roman Bones
by Clair C. Patterson

The Roman bones submitted by S. C. Gilfillan to the California Institute of Technology, Division of Geological and Planetary Sciences, for lead analyses by C. Patterson and E. Bingham were contaminated by soil that had been in contact with the bones in the presence of moisture for centuries. The soil removed from the bones by sonic treatment was analyzed for lead, so that for each bone sample two lead analyses were available: that in bone and that in soil attached to the bone. Each bone sample contained small amounts of soil particles that remained attached to the bone after cleaning. The amount of residual particle soil lead in each bone sample was determined from an aluminum analysis. The

182

aluminum content was multiplied by the Pb/Al ratio in the sonically isolated soil to obtain a soil particle lead content of the bone that was subtracted from the total lead found in the bone.

Since ionic, or soluble, lead in the soil had also been absorbed by the bone and incorporated chemically into the calcium phosphate phase of the bone, some method had to be devised for estimating this chemically absorbed ionic soil lead in each bone so that it could be subtracted from the total bone lead. Lead concentrations in sonically isolated soil from Roman bones ranged from 10 to 2,800 ppm; but the average concentration of lead in soil contacting the vertebrae and long bones of the Roman poor was 180 ppm, which was considerably less than the average of 720 ppm lead in soil contacting the vertebrae and long bones of the Roman rich. The greater average total lead content in bones of the rich (190 ppm) compared to that in the bones of the poor (50 ppm) might therefore have resulted, in part, from a greater absorption of ionic lead from greater amounts of lead in soil contacting the bones of the rich. These averages are only for vertebrae and long bones analyzed at LCIT that have been corrected for residual soil particle lead, age, and type of bone. They should not be mistaken for Gilfillan's final averages.

Total bone leads, minus soil particle leads, in 18 bones from Roman poor were plotted as a function of lead in soil, as shown in Figure A, on the next page. The graph points were divided arbitrarily into two populations: those whose bone lead contents were determined by soil lead concentrations, and those whose bone lead contents were independent of soil lead concentrations. The demarcation between these two populations starts at the zero origin, and it is believed that the amount of lead that bone absorbs chemically from the soil increases with increasing lead in soil to a situation where approximately 200 ppm lead in soil contributes about 40 ppm chemically absorbed lead in bone. Greater amounts of lead in soil are not believed to contribute much more lead to bone, because tenfold increases in concentrations of lead in soil do not seem to add any more lead to bone. In order to be conservative and make a maximum correction for chemically absorbed soil lead, a smooth curve was drawn thru the highest bone-lead concentrations in the population of data points assumed to be determined by soil lead concentrations. Only one-third of the bone samples of the Roman poor were therefore found to contain lead in excess of that which was probably contributed by chemical absorption from soil. The curve shown in Figure A was used to correct total bone leadings in the poor for chemically absorbed soil lead. Starting with the concentration of lead in the dirt associated with a given bone, a corresponding value obtained from the curve in Figure A for the amount of lead chemically absorbed from the soil in that bone was found. This quantity of chemically absorbed

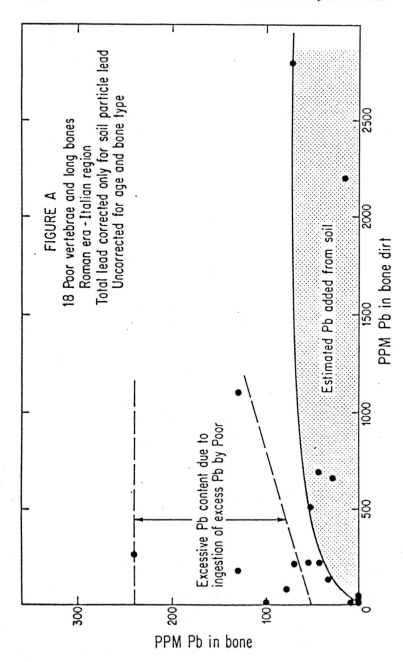

FIGURE A

18 Poor vertebrae and long bones
Roman era - Italian region
Total lead corrected only for soil particle lead
Uncorrected for age and bone type

Excessive Pb content due to
ingestion of excess Pb by Poor

Estimated Pb added from soil

PPM Pb in bone dirt

PPM Pb in bone

soil lead was then subtracted from the total amount of lead found in the bone. This correction varied with the amount of lead in the soil contacting the bone, and in 11 out of 18 cases it accounted for essentially all of the lead found in the bone.

Since the same factors that generated the soil lead relations in the bones of the poor also operated in the same fashion on the bones of the rich, the curve in Figure A was also used to correct total bone leadings in the rich for chemically absorved soil lead. The new averages, after this type of correction, were 44 ppm (50 ppm uncorrected) lead in bones of the Roman poor and 155 ppm (190 ppm uncorrected) lead in the bones of the Roman rich. The difference between the rich and the poor therefore probably did not result from a difference in lead absorbed from soil. These numbers should not be mistaken for Gilfillan's final averages.

180 ppm lead in soil is about twentyfold above natural levels, and since there are no geochemical reasons for presuming otherwise, this excess lead is probably anthropogenic. It is not known whether this lead had been introduced recently or in ancient times, but it is likely that a significant portion is ancient. This lead is absorbed on the surfaces of clays and is chelated by humic acids; it is relatively mobile in the sense that it can be transferred to other powerful chelating surfaces such as calcium phosphate thru an aqueous medium during centuries of time. 44 ppm lead observed in average dry Roman poor bones is close to the observed present average value of 33 ppm lead in dry American bones,[1] but these values are hundreds of times greater than the natural levels of about 0.1 ppm lead in dry human prehistoric bones, estimated from the biodiminution of lead in natural food chains.[2]

Gilfillan submitted three different samples of human bones taken from the Italian region (including Sardinia) that were dated at 1000 to 2000 B.C. These bones contained about 2 ppm Pb, on the average, but they also contained about 25 percent by weight of soil clay. If the clay contained 8 ppm or more lead, the dry bones would contain considerably less than 1 ppm lead after a correction only for soil particle lead. A correction would still be needed for chemically absorbed soil lead. Gilfillan also submitted a sample of human bone from a Central Egyptian rich mummy dated at 200 B.C. This bone contained 1 ppm lead, but no soil, nor had it been in contact with soil. It was blackened from the embalming resin, however, and may have absorbed some lead from that substance. (Lead products were freely used in the culture at that time.) I. M. Shapiro and co-workers have found similar concentrations of lead in the teeth of Egyptian mummies that were a thousand years older,[3] but still, in those cultures artifact lead products were commonly used by the rich.

Shapiro and co-workers actually found 0.3 ppm lead in bones (converted from secondary dentine values) of primitive Indians living in a remote region of Mexico,[4] but these persons were exposed to significant amounts of industrial artifact lead in their food and air, from lead solder and leaded aerosols.

Ericson, Shirahata, and Patterson have observed an interesting relation between lead in tooth enamel and lead in bone from protoceramic culture humans buried in dry Peruvian soil for 4,000 years.[5] In this case tooth enamel contained 0.2 ppm lead, while dry femur bone free of soil particles contained 1.0 ppm lead. In a living person the lead concentrations in tooth enamel is about 1.3 times greater than in bone. It is obvious that the concentration of chemically absorbed soil lead is far greater in the more porous bone of the skeleton than in denser, less porous tooth enamel. More than 80 percent of the 1 ppm lead found in the protoceramic bone was chemically absorbed from soil containing 10 ppm of lead. The bones were retrieved from a mound in a desert where the rainfall was 0.3 cm/yr. It is not yet known what fraction of the 0.2 ppm lead in the protoceramic tooth enamel was chemically absorbed from soil, but it is clear that the original lead content of this material is very close to the natural lead 0.1 ppm estimated from the biodiminution of lead in natural food chains.

This means that the Roman poor were also subjected to a form of lead poisoning, called severe chronic lead insult,[6] which was milder than that experienced by the noble class of Romans in that it would not result in a high incidence of overt infertility and madness. Nevertheless, it is believed that this severe chronic insult form of lead poisoning, which also affects most Americans today, did cause increased mental irritability, reduced mental acuity, reduced resistance to disease, and damaged germ plasm in the Roman poor. The per capita production of lead in Roman times was about one-fifth of that in today's industrialized regions.[7] In terms of significant poisonous effects on the main segment of human populations thruout time, lead is probably the world's most ancient environmental poison, extending back in time for thousands of years.

The Presentation of the Bone Analyses
by S. Colum Gilfillan

For our present reporting, the bones (and a few other objects also assayed for lead) have been first divided into six groups according to the periods and areas covered and the significance of their data, groups labeled A to F. The first groups are the most significant for our thesis.

Within each group the bones are first designated by their analysis number, and often subgrouped according to the museum and/or personal donor, to whom go our sincere thanks. Then we state in successive order the place and date of death, the surroundings if known and significant (for example, a tomb), the sex if known, which bone of the body, the analyzing laboratory (L), the amounts of other poisonous metals if found, then the lead found, each in milligrams per kilogram of *dried* bone, counted as ppm and often corrected for dirt in the bone (CD); then CB, the correction of the lead figure by the Which-bone Factor; then the person's age, if known (if unknown, assumed to be an adult); then the correction, if any, for the person's age, CA; and last his social status R (rich), MC (middle class), or P (poor). The student should especially compare our last lead measure available and stated, as related to the person's social status, country, and era, whether we have been able to refine our findings more, or less, by facts supplied by the donor, or by the laboratory. Items omitted were not available.

At the conclusion of Group A, which is restricted to bones of known social class, from the Roman Empire in space and time, the averages of leading are computed for the three main classes: Rich, Middle Class, and Poor. And for this group, as for each of the other five groups, the total of cases is counted; but averages have been computed only for Group A. The studious reader can readily compile his own further averages as he thinks fit.

The method we think best for computing the three class averages for that most important Group A, from the Roman Empire, we have discussed in Chapter 8. There we tell how we deal with the important age factor, as well as the piling up of lead, chiefly in the shaft bones, where it is almost harmless but whose existence proves prior poisoning on its way from mouth or lung to long bone, perhaps with a stop-off in a porous bone.

Many unused portions of the LCIT bones are preserved, but not those from the Kettering Laboratory; and some bones and objects preserved were not assayed. Inquiries, from serious scientists only, should be addressed to the Smithsonian Institution, Washington, D.C.

1.   H. A. Schroeder and I. H. Tipton. The human body burden of lead. *Archives of Env. Health*, 17:965-978 (1968).
2.   R. Elias, Y. Hirao, and C. Patterson. Impact of present levels of aerosol Pb concentrations on both natural ecosystems and humans. *International Conference on Heavy Metals in the Environment*, Toronto, Oct. 1975, Vol. 2, Part 1, pp. 257-272.

3.   I. M. Shapiro, G. Mitchell, I. Davidson and S. H. Katz. The lead content of teeth. *Archives of Env. Health*, 30:483-486 (1975).

4.   J. Ericson, H. Shirahata, and C. Patterson. Skeletal concentrations of lead in ancient Peruvians: *New England J. of Medicine*, 100:946-951 (1979).

5.   C. Patterson. Contaminated and natural lead environments of man. *Archives of Env. Health*, 11:356 (1965).

6.   C. Patterson. Silver stocks and losses in Ancient and Medieval times. *Economic Hist. Rev.*, 2nd series, 25:205-235 (1972).

7.   Some scientists elsewhere have given the proportions of lead in terms of the raw, wet bone, or of the ashed bone. Such measurements can be approximately converted to our own dry bone standard by the following formulae: the proportion of lead in ashed bone would be 1.67 times its proportion in dry bone, the proportion in fresh bone would be one-third of the dry proportion, and for fresh teeth about nine-tenths. F. Weyrauch and H. Muller: Distribution of lead in blood, organs and bones [in German], *Zeitschrift fur Hyg. Infekt. Kr.*, 115:216-20, 1933. Or see G. H. Hansmann and M. C. Perry: Lead Absorption and Intoxication, *Archives of Pathology* (Chicago), 30:226-35, 1940.

Appendix B

Bones Assayed

Following are the abbreviations used in this appendix.

A.D.   Anno Domini (in the year of Our Lord). The first century of the Christian era.

Ag   silver content, in ppm (parts per million)

bnv   but not very

ca.   approximately

CA   corrected to take account of the person's age

CB   corrected for which-bone, showing how much lead it would most likely have held, had it been a rib.

CD   the leading, corrected for dirt in it.

Cd   cadmium content in ppm

Cu   copper content in ppm

F   female

LCIT   analyzed spectrographically at the California Institute of Technology in Pasadena, in 1973-74, under the direction of Prof. Clair C. Patterson, thru the hand of Elizabeth Bingham.

LKK   analyzed by the Kettering Laboratory of the University of Cincinnati, in 1964, under Dr. Robert A. Kehoe, using the dithizone colorimetric method primarily, sometimes supplemented by the spectrographic method.

LKY   analyzed by the Kettering Laboratory, in 1975, under Prof. David W. Yeager, using the spectrographic method.

M   male

MC   middle class

n.c.   not corrected

P   poor

Pb   lead content in ppm

ppm   parts per million, by weight of dried bone

prob.   probably

R   rich

Sn   tin content in ppm

Zn   zinc content in ppm

189

Our procedures have been explained and our general rationale and findings given in Chapter 8. The totals of bones and people listed in each group below are given at its end. The median average leadings are computed for Group A only. The first letters and numbers listed for each item are the donor's identification number for that specimen.

Group A: Bones from the Roman Empire, 150 B.C. to 476 A.D., and Identifiable by Social Class

Rome

The directors of the great Museo Nazionale delle Terme in Rome were especially helpful. Dottoressa Eleonora Bracco gave me in 1963 the following seven bones, presumably from Rome or its vicinity. All of these, except the last one, have been analyzed by LCIT.

G Br 2   ca. 280 A.D., porous end of a long bone; Cu 21; CD 400; CB 500?; rich freedwoman or freeborn; R.

G Br 1c   jawbone; Cu 86; CD 130; CB 65; prob. P.

G Br 3a   third century A.D.; left jawbone, back end; Cu 26; Pb 44 (not corrected for dirt); CB 22; P. Also Dr. Irving M. Shapiro kindly tested the dentine of a canine tooth from the above jaw and found 68 ppm, not a heavy leading; CB 21; P.

G Br 3b   ca. 390 A.D., Christian; femur, prob. shaft; Cu 10; CD 79; CB 33; P.

G Br 1b   lower end of R. femur shaft; F; Cu 6; CD 71; CB 30; prob. P.

G Br 1a   F; R. femur shaft; CD 29; CB 14; P bnv.

2000   M; sternum; LKK; Pb 151; CB 73; young adult, if 20 then his CA should be 158; R.

From the same great Museum in Rome the successor Director, Elisa Coronna Lissi, gave me the following three bones in 1972, analyzed by LCIT.

G Ro-1   2nd century A.D.; from ceramic coffin; R. rib; Cu 50; CD 210; "a girl," if age were 8, CA would be 676, P bnv.

G Ro 124735 young person from marble coffin; vertebra side spine; Cu 49; CD 86; CB 63; CA for age 20 would be 136; R.

G Ro 128577 from marble coffin; femur, top of shaft; Cu 40; CD 330; CB 138; R.

2006   Mr. Jones of the Instituto Brittanica, near Rome, gave me the following bone from Rosso della Crescrenza near Rome, from 2nd-3rd century A.D.; tile grave; F; metacarpus of index finger; LKK; Pb 213; CB 1030; age 45; P bnv.

Vatican City

The following five bones were given to me in 1963 by Prof. Magi from a Christian cemetery of about the 2nd century A.D. The bones were discovered in Vatican City when excavation was in progress for a modern garage. Those buried there were said to have been poor, but some seemed to me middle class; but call all P bnv; all analyzed by LKK.

2004   palate; Pb 95; CB as jaw 47.5; age 9; CA 675; P bnv.
2003   bone unidentified; 2nd century A.D.; Pb 82; P bnv.
2006   part of long bone, near end; Pb 91; CB 110; P bnv.
2002   vertebra; Pb 125.6; CB 92; P bnv.
2001   skull or scapula; Pb 46.5; CB 36?; P bnv.

Florence

The following two bones were given to me by Edoardo Pardini of the Istuto di Antropol. in Florence and were analyzed by LCIT. They came from a tomb of the Licinii Crassi family, on the Appian Way near Rome, of the first or second century A.D.

GR 3808   F; side knob of vertebra; little dirt; Cu 150; Sn 69; Ag 3; CD 110; CB 80; R.
GR 3815 bis   F; sid knob of vertebra; Cu in dirt more than 300; CD 330; R.

Viterbo

The following three bones were also given to me by Edoardo Pardini and came from the Tomb of the Shepherds in Viterbo, Lazio, north of Rome. They are from the third to fourth century A.D., all vertebrae. The central spine was examined, and all were analyzed by LCIT.

GVGS+   M; Cu 6; Ag 2; CD 100; CB 73; age 30; CA 98; P.
GVGS-O   M; Cu 10; CD 10; age 30; CA 14.7; P.
GVGS-A   F; Cu 36; CD 250; CB 183; over 40?; P.

Sicily

GA 2   Agrigento, Sicily, Villa Aurea necropolis; Christian; 4th
            century A.D.; from a tomb dug in a rock; scapula, joint
            end; LKY; Pb 33.4; CB 20; R.
GA 1a   Agrigento; 4th century A.D.; Christian; from a catacomb;
            curved tubular small bone, prob. clavicle; LKY; Pb 25.7;
            CB 19.3; prob. MC.

Tunisia

T-1   el Djem, Tunisia, ancient Thysdrus; 2nd-3rd century
            A.D.; possibly cremated; rib fragments and teeth, assume
            former analyzed; LKK; a small person, perhaps not full
            grown, but of a small race; Pb 73.1; R.

Sardinia

The following five bones (as well as 2 in Group B and 27 in Group D),
were given to me by Prof. Carlo Maxia, Director of the Institute of
Anthropol. Sciences at the University of Cagliari, Sardinia, and were
analyzed by LCIT.

GC-22   from the Old Christian Cemetery, Cornus in Sardinia;
            3rd century A.D.; lower jaw; Cu 31; CD 55; CB 27; prob.
            lower MC because Christian.
GC-23   same cemetery; 3rd century A.D.; upper jaw?; Cu 30;
            CD 79; CB 34.1; prob. lower MC because Christian.
GC-15   Roman era; Cagliari, Sardinia, from a tomb; tibia shaft;
            Cu 10; CD 23; CB 11; R.
GC-16   prob. from a Roman tomb; no date; femur shaft; Cu 5;
            CD 2; CB 0.84; R?
GC-17   Roman period; from a tomb; prob. femur shaft; Cu 4;
            CD 13; CB 6.8; R?

Belgrad

Marko Popovíc of the Muzej Grada Beograda, Belgrad, very kindly sent
me the following nine valuable bones, beside others not analyzed, from
three ancient people in 1968. The following analyses were made by
LCIT.
    From Belgrad, ancient Singidunum in the province of Dalmatia, from
the Roman necropolis on Kosovska Street, four bones from a lady of

the mid-third century A.D., from a well-done sarcophagus containing golden jewelry, were analyzed. Perhaps she died of lead poisoning, which had piled up faster in her more porous bones than in her femus and skull. Also analyzed were three bones from a baby, and a bone and tooth from a 17-year-old young woman.

While we have had analyzed, and report below, each of the eight bones and a tooth, we have put into our general averages for Group A only one measure, an average, for each of the three different individuals (three measures from nine analyses).

GB I/1	a F of 15-20 years of age from whom the following 4 bones were analyzed; skull part with 2% of dirt; Cu 76; Pb 120 n.c. for dirt; CB 93; CA 208; R.
GB I/3	same girl; vertebra; Ag 1; Cu 47; Pb 150 n.c.; CB 109; CA 240; R.
GB I/4	same girl; pelvic trough; Cu 210; Pb 190 n.c.; CB 143; CA 250; R.
GB I/5	same girl; femur; Cu 20; Pb 100 n.c.; CB 42; CA 112; her average 202.5; R.
GB II/1	Baby of 1 yr. prob. of same family; skull; Cu 57; CD 170; CB 132; CA 1720 fatal; R.
GB II/2	same baby; rib; Cu over 400; Pb 730 n.c.; CA 9600 fatal; R.
GB II/3	same baby; femur, end?; Cu 120; Pb 89 in dirt; Pb in bone 200; CB 250; CA 3300 fatal; baby's average 4873; R.
GB III/1	from a small tomb 10 km. from Belgrad, painted red inside; 3rd or 4th century A.D.; F; skull; Cu 3; Pb 30 n.c.; CB 26.8; age ca. 17; CA 53; MC?
GB III/2	a pre-molar tooth from same young woman was analyzed by Dr. Irving M. Shapiro who found 41.03 ppm Pb; CB 18.8, a low leading; MC?

Britain

We may recall that the climate of Britain has rarely permitted the growing of grapes, especially in northern Britain; so wines and grape syrup would be expensive. But lead was abundant.

The following six bones from York, probably from later Roman centuries, were given to me by Professor Roger Warwick of Guy's Hospital, London, in 1962; they were analyzed for lead only by LKK. All were poor.

307 A   scapula; Pb 37; CB 27.8; P.
601   M; manubrium sterni; Pb 44;3; CB 22?; P.
460   M; scapula; Pb 30.4; CB 23.1; age 35; CA 26; P.
471-1   M; scapula; Pb 46.7; CB 35.1; age 25; CA 76; P.
424   scapula; Pb 11.7; CB 8.8; P.
610   F; prob. jaw; Pb 54.4; CB 27; age 35; CA 63; P.

The following six bones were given to me in 1963 by Dr. K. P. Oakley
of the British Museum (Natural History), London, and were analyzed by
LKK.

4.135   from Eaton; 1st century A.D.; scapula; Pb 14.9; CB 12.2;
             MC?
4.10.10   from Compton Abdale; in a stone coffin; 3rd to 4th
             century A.D.; adult F; scapula; Pb 41.6; CB 31; R.
11;53   scapula from York, prob. F; Pb 16; CB 12; P.
4.1702   from Landsdown, Brockham End, 2nd century A.D.;
             sternum; M; Pb 12.9; CB 6.2; age 30-40; CA 7.3; R.
4.1389   M; sternum; Pb 81; CB 39.3; age 30-40; CA 49.3; P.
1956.29.7.1 from a grain pit; prob. F; scapula; Pb 1.6; CB 1.2; P.

Don R. Brothwell, of the Britiah Museum (Natural History) kindly gave
me the following two bones in 1973; analyzed at LKY.

Anc 184,   from Ancaster, Lincolnshire; A.D. 375; vertebra; Pb 82;
  1968   CB 59.6; lower MC.
Anc 119a,   375 A.D.; M; vertebra; Pb 12.8; CB 9.3; lower MC.
  1966

Emporion (presumed lead workers)

The following ten bones analyzed from nine people (beside three
others from ancient northeastern Hispania which we shall list in Group
C) were given to the author by Dr. Maria de los Dolores del Amo Guinovart of the Archeological Museum of Tarragone, Spain. The nine people came from the Pere Martell cemetery, dating from A.D. 250-400,
near the ancient fortified seaport city Emporion, modern Ampurias, at
the northeasternmost tip of Spain. Founded by Greeks from Massilia
(Marseille), the city was not very far from lead and silver mines, and
doubtless shipped and probably fashioned leaden wares and ingots.
Such occupations apparently put lead into the air and soil as well as into
the workers, whose bones had an almost uniformly very high leading,
averaging 249. So these Emporion workers could serve as samples of

the ancient lead-working poor, but not of the Roman poor in general. So we should not put all the lead weight of all of them into our average for the universal Roman poor class, but use them as an extensive example of the lead-working poor, tho their very air and ground were drenched with that and other poisonous metals. The donor, De. Guinovart, classed them all socially as "poor, but not very" (P bnv). Their average leading, corrected for intrusive posthumous dirt, which had entraordinary quantities of the poisonous metals copper (Cu) and silver (Ag), indicating that both their work and their soil were industrially poisoned. All these bones were analyzed by LCIT.

GAM 5 (11)	rib; Cu 72; Pb in dirt 420; Pb in bone 150 n.c.; age ca. 7; CA 940; P bnv.
GSPT 23 (22)-1	ulna?; Cu 72; Pb in dirt 2800?; CD 73; CB 40; P bnv.
GSPT 23 (22)-2	prob. same person; vertebra; Cu 92; Ag 3; CD 240; CB 175. We shall count only the average CB for the 2 bones, P bnv.
GET 28 (33)	femur shaft, Cu 14 n.c.; Pb in dirt 510; CD 53; CB 91.4; age ca. 17; CA 56.5; Pbnv.
GSP 2 (6)	vertebra; Ag 8, Cu 160; Pb 280 n.c. for lead in dirt, which was 460; CB 205; age ca. 17; CA 525?; P bnv.
GTAR 18 (8)	rib; Cu 200; CD 190; P bnv.
GE 15 B	adult vertebra; Cu 110 n.c.; Ag 4 n.c.; Pb 190 before corrections for dirt that contained 420; CB 205; P bnv
GE 11 (12)	vertebra; Cu 93; Ag 7; Pb 250 n.c.; CB 182; P bnv.
GAM 1 (3)	rib; Cu 100; Pb 130 n.c.; Pb in dirt 320; age ca. 5; CA 566; P bnv.
GSP 15 A	F; femur, upper epiphysis; Cu 150; CD 240; CB 300; P bnv.

Totals and Averages for Group A

46 people were analyzed for Group A, beside 6 additional bones analyzed from 3 of these people, for a total of 52 bones. These exclude Emporion's poor lead workers.

Our social class averages, computed from their class medians (for the reason explained in Chapter 8 which is to avoid undue weighting by a few individuals who have an overkill dose of lead, especially young people computed according to their age factor), show rationalized, *median* average leadings of 80 ppm of lead in our 15 rich people, 27 ppm as the median average for our 7 middle-class folk, and 34.5 ppm as the median average for our 24 poor, excluding the Emporion group.

Those 10 *Emporion* bones from 9 people in the lead-working town, all poor bnv., had a median average of 205. If it be proper (as the writer inclines to think) to include in our Empire's poor median average 1 or possibly 2 Emporion average (median) cases, to represent the unquestionably numerous lead workers among the ancient poor, this would take the Empire's poor median average to 36 with the addition of one Emporion median case, or to 42.6 with the addition of 2 Emporions.

Group B; Outside the Empire in Place or Time, and Identifiable by Social Class

72AA	from the Agora of Athens in an 8th century B.C. cemetery, in a tomb; an unidentified bone; LKK; Pb 41.3; R.
2007	from Jones of the British Academy in Rome in 1963, from Villanova near Rome; 8-7th century B.C.; prob. a shaft bone; LKK; Pb 19.4; CB 9?; P.
G RA (2)	from the Museum in Ragusa, Sicily, from Castiglione; 6th century B.C.; from a tomb; LCIT; rib of a child; Pb 1; R.
G Ra-2	from the Museum in Ragusa, Sicily; from a tomb; 3rd or 4th century B.C.; LCIT; vertebra; Cu 13; CD less than 10; prob. R.
Egypt	middle area, ca. 200 B.C.; given by M. F. Gaballah and I. M. Kamel; solid portion of the vertebra of a mummy were analyzed in LCIT by isotope dilution mass spectrometry, the very best method; Pb only 1 ppm; R.
GC-21	Cagliari, Bithia-Tombe, Punic-Roman from Prof. Maxia; 500-238 B.C.; from a tomb; tibia shaft; LCIT; Cu 2; CD 34; CB 16; prob. R.
GC-18	Dolianova, Lombard medieval, A.D. 574-774; from a tomb; M; clavicle, LCIT; Cu 5; CD 2; prob. R.
GC-19	Lombard medieval; from Dolianova, Sardinia, and with the two items above from Prof. Maxia; from a Lombard tomb; clavicle; LCIT; Cu 5; CD 1; prob. R.

Group B Total: 8 bones and people

Group C: From the Empire, but Not Identifiable by Social Class

AC 35	from Ancaster, Britain, 1965 excavations; rib; LCIT; Pb 49.7.
GA-4	from Basel, Helvetia; 4th century A.D.; rib; LKK; Pb

30.3.

The following three bones were given to me by Dr. Guinovart from the Emporion collection described at the end of Group A. But their origins named appear to be other localities in northeastern Hispania. So we place them here and cannot be sure of their social class. All were analyzed by LCIT.

GE 23   from Tercio de Montserrat, a cemetery outside Barcelona; very small rib of a child; Cu 110; CD 140; CA 1000?

GE 35   vertebra from Tercio de Montserrat; Cu 47; Ag 4; CD 45; CB 33.

GE 8 (13)   from Campiona ig Dolianova; combined top and shaft of a prob. fibula; LCIT; Pb in dirt 1100?; Cu 57; CD 130; CB 210

Group C Total: 5 bones and people.

Group D: Outside the Empire in Time or Space and Not Identifiable by Social Class

The following three bones from Castiglione in the sixth century B.C. were received from the Museum in Ragusa, Sicily, and were analyzed by LCIT.

G Ra 122   vertebra; Cu 25; CD 1.

G Ra (2)   two children's or a child's ribs; Cu 42 or 48; Pb 1.

G Ra T 101   from a tomb with several skeletons; vertebra; Cu 50; Pb 3; R?

The following five bones are from the Agora, the marketplace of Athens, and were given me by the American School of Classical Studies there, chiefly thru the kindness of Dr. J. Lawrence Angel in 1967, Curator of Physical Anthropology in the Smithsonian Institution in Washington, D.C., and by others thru correspondence; and thru Nathaniel Weyl. All were analyzed by LKK in 1964.

61 AA   700-550 B.C.; phalanx; Pb 62; CB 29.

70 AA   550-525 B.C.; which bone not known; Pb 35.

69 AA   before 500 B.C.; which bone not known; Pb 226.

19 AA   A.D. 400-500; which bone not known; Pb 28.2.

180 AA   A.D. 1450-1825; Turkish era; which bone not known;

Pb 117.

The following bones were kindly provided by Prof. Carlo Maxia of the University of Cagliari, who also paid part of the cost of analyzing some of these bones by LKY.

GC-1-C	from Alghero, Grotto naturale "de lu maccioni"; Neolithic age; ulna shaft; LCIT; Cu 31; CD 2; CB 1.1?
GC-2-CT	same place; neolithic; femur shaft; LCIT; Cu 2; CD 4; CB 1.7?
GC-3	same place; neolithic; humerus distal epiphysis, shaft analyzed; LCIT; Cu 2; CD 3; CB 2?
GCa 21	Cagliari; eneolithic (bronze & stone) age; cranium; LKY; Pb 510; CB 395.
GCa 23	Cagliari; eneolithic; cranium; LKY; Pb 954; CB 753.
CR 7	Cagliari from San Benedetto; eneolithic; 6th cent. B.C. or earlier; leaded prob. from spring water; cranium; LKY; Pb 328; CB 254.
GCa 20	Cagliari; eneolithic; cranium; LKY; Pb 452; CB 350.
CR 1	Cagliari; eneolithic; 6th century B.C. or earlier; cranium I; LKY; Pb 343; CB 265.
GC-7	from San Benedetto (Iglesias); eneolithic; femur shaft; LCIT; Cu 4; CD 53; CB 22?
GC-8	from Cerra Crabiles (Sennori Osib); eneolithic; femur top; LCIT; Cu 8; CD 2; CB 2.5?
GCa 19	eneolithic; cranium; LKY; Pb 318; CB 246.
GC-4	Villa Massargia; eneolithic; humerus shaft; LCIT; Cu 18; Ag 4; Zn 840; CD 13; CB 8.4?
GC-6	San Benedetto; eneolithic; tibia shaft; LCIT; Zn and Cd very heavy; Ag 1; Cu 4; CD 56; CB 79.
GC-5	Villa Massargia; eneolithic; manubrium sterni; LCIT; Cu 11; CD 310; CB 150.
GC-9	from Cerra Crabiles (Sennori Osib); eneolithic; metatarsal from foot; LCIT; Cu 11; Ag 2; CD 3; CB 14?
GCa 4	Cagliari; eneolithic; cranium; LKY; Pb 664; CB 515.
GCa 6	Cagliari; drank from a leaded spring; cranium; LKY; Pb 275; CB 213.
GC-10	Sevio; from the nuragic era, which extended from ca. 1000 B.C. to 490 B.C.; ulna shaft; LCIT; Cu 3; CD 2; CB 1.4.
GC-11	Sevio; nuragic era; radius; LCIT; Cu 10; CD 1; CB 1.2.
GC-14a	Sevio; Capo Pecora (Fumini maggiore); nuragic; femur shaft; LCIT; Cu 2; Ag 2; CD 9; CB 3.8.

GC-14b	Sevio; Capo Pecora (Fumini maggiore); nuragic; same person as 14a and same bone; prox. epiphysis; LCIT; CD 21. The marked difference between the lead ratings of the two parts of the same bone is probably due to the lead going first into the porous epiphysis, then gradually collecting in the dense shaft.
GC-12	Perdas de fogo (Grotta funerara); nuragic; clavicle; LCIT; Cu 28; CD 27.
GC-13	Matrox e bois (Usellus) Poliandro; nuragic Roman; femur prox. epiphysis; LCIT; Cu 58; CD 19; CB 24.
GC-20	Cagliari; Punic Roman; radius shaft; LCIT; Cu 46; CD 4; CB 2.3
GC-25	Tharros, Old Christian cemetery; 6-7th century A.D.; tibia; LCIT; Cu 4; CD 14; CB 6.4.
GC-24	Tharros, same cemetery; 6th-7th century A.D.; humerus; LCIT; Cu 15; Ag 1; CD 65; CB 42.

Group D Totals: 34 bones from 33 people.

Group E: Bones Analyzed but Not Fully Calculated Because of Some Abnormality Named, Usually Cremation or Being in a Well

GY-2	Zadar, Yugoslavia; A.D. 20-30 cemetery; cremated; rib; LCIT; Cu 6; Pb 4 n.c.; lower MC.
GY-1	from same cemetery and time; cremated; vertebra; LCIT; Cu 7; Pb 5 n.c.; CB 3.6; lower MC.
V-2	Mostar, Yugoslavia; 1st-3rd century A.D.; in urn; dirty, cremated; cranium and metatarsal or metacarpus; LKK; Pb 15.3; P.
V-1	Vukodol, Yugoslavia; 1st century A.D.; in urn; cremated, dirty; fibula; LKK; Pb 4.33; CB 5.1; R.
G Po	Pompeii; tomb; cremated; vertebra; LCIT; Cu 31; CD 71; CB 52; R.
G Si	Syracuse; bronze urn; cremated; vertebra; LCIT; copper a major element; CD 24; CB 17.5; prob. R.
G Pa Ma	Marsala, ancient Lilybaeum, Sicily; 2nd century B.C.; cremated; tubular bone; LCIT; Cu 7; CD 16.

Prof. Fouet of the University of Toulouse sent the following two bones from Roman Gaul. They were also analyzed by Dr. Ralph E. Nusbaum.

GB-1	Beaugou (Corrèze) France; 3rd-4th century A.D.; crema-

ted; misc. bones including epistropheum vertebra; LKK;
Pb 8; CB 6; P.

OB-3   Leyssène (Corrèze) France; 1st century A.D.; cremated;
                  jaw; LKK; Pb 23.1; CB 11.5; R.

G Cy   Salamis, Cyprus; 8th century B.C.; bronze urn in royal
                  tomb; cremated; F; small tubular bone of hand or foot;
                  LCIT; Cu 370 n.c. for dirt; Pb 3 n.c.; CB 14; R.

G Ra 101   Ragusa, Sicily; 6th century B.C.; prob. cremated; rib;
                  LCIT; Pb 1; a child; R.

G Ra 2   Ragusa, Sicily (Cortalilio); 5th-4th century B.C.; tomb;
                  may be cremated; vertebra; LCIT; Pb less than 10; prob.
                  R.

G Ra 122-1   Ragusa, Sicily (Castiglione); 6th century B.C.; tomb;
                  prob. cremated; rib; LCIT; Pb ca. 1; a child; prob. R.

The following ten bones from nine people came from excavations in
the Agora, the marketplace of ancient Athens, thru the very helpful
services as those in Group D, but these came from *wells*, so we have not
trusted their leading not to have been contaminated by lead pails or
other leaden objects lost in the well.

AA 77   1st to 4th century A.D.; pelvis; LCIT; Cu over 400; CD
                  270; CB 202, age 8; CA 820.

AA 79   7th century A.D.; pelvis; LCIT; much Cu; Pb 480 n.c.;
                  CB 362; age 5; CA 1562.

14 AA   1st century A.D.; LKK; Pb 300.

AA 78   ca. A.D. 625; fibula end; LCIT; Cu 220; Pb in dirt 43; in
                  bone 410; age 5; much Cu.

13 AA   1st century A.D.; rib?; LKK; Pb 86.4.

10 AA   400 B.C.; LKK; Pb 86.4

24 AA   90 B.C.; LKK; Pb 492.

20 AA   400-500 A.D.; LKK; Pb 568.

76 AA   2nd-4th century A.D.; M; rib; LKK; Pb 391; age 32; CA
                  463.

AA 76   same M as above; rib; LCIT; Cu 170; CD 210; CA 344.

(The minor discrepancy between the above two measurements by the
two laboratories was doubtless due partly to their assaying different
parts of the same rib. Large differences occur between the lead content of the dense exterior and the porous interior of a rib. And LKK
had only three-fourths of a gram of bone.)

4.1385   Chester, Britain; F; pelvis; LKK; age 21; Pb 6140, too much.

1956.24. from S. Cerney, Gloucester; 150-200 A.D.; in a lead coffin;
10.1 F; scapula; LKK; age 45; Pb 258; R.

Group E Totals: 25 bones from 24 people.

Group F/ Assays of Objects Other than Bones

The following samples of dirt from amphoras were analyzed by LKY.

GC-1 from the Museum of Crotone, Calabria, Capo Colonna; hard clumps of dirt; Pb 11.7.

GC-2 from the same place; finer dust; Pb 14.8.

GC-3 from the same place; from shipwreck; Pb 97.2.

0-38420 Shells from shipwrecked amphora near Bitia, Sardinia; given by the Romisch-Germanisches Zentralmuseum in Mainz; Pb 14.4.

Pom-1 Garum (fish sauce); said to be ancient when given to the author in Pompeii; dry, clear solid gelatin, good tasting; Pb 39.5.

Pom-2 Dirt removed by the author from inside a recently discovered amphora in Pompeii; Pb 33.1. (See Plate 6 on page 70.)

Group F Totals: 6 objects.

Appendix C

Which-Bone Factor for Lead

| Bone Pair | Direct Ratio to Rib | | |
	Weighted Average Ratio	No. of Pairs	Separate Studies Combined
Vertebra/rib	1.37	168	12
Femur/rib	2.38	60	6
Femur end/rib	.80	1	
Cranium/rib	1.29	1071	
Petrous temporal bone/rib	1.94	41	
Tibia/rib	2.14	81	6
Tibia endpiece/rib	.84	1	
Tibia shaft/rib	.71	1	
Radius shaft/rib	.83	1	
Radius end/rib	1.65	1	
Fibula shaft/rib	.84	1	
Jaw/rib	2.00	9	
Teeth/rib	2.18	16	2

Indirect Ratios, based on First bone/Other-bone-named ratio.

Humerus/rib	1.55	4	Humerus/vertebra 1.13
Sternum/rib	2.00	1	Sternum/long bones 2.0
Ulna/rib	1.84	1	Ulna/cranium 1.39
Talus/rib	.49	1	Talus/vertebra .58
Phalanx/rib	.21	1	Phalanx/vertebra .28
Pelvis/rib, or Scapula/rib	1.33	0	Having found no bone-pairs for these, we assign to them the average rib ratio of the similarly porous bones, the vertebra and cranium.

Sources for Which-Bone Data

C. Badham and H. B. Taylor: from an Australian report cited by Cantarow, Ab., and Max Trumper*: *Lead Poisoning*, 1944, 6th ed., 1962, pub. by Saunders of Phila., p. 240, and Table 6, p. 29.

P. S. I. Barry: A Comparison of Lead Concentrations in Human Bones and in Soft Tissues: *Amsterdam International Symposium on Environmental Lead*, 1972.

B. T. Emmerson and D. S. Lecky: The Lead Content of Bone in Subjects without recognized past exposure and in patients with renal disease. *Australian Annals of Medicine.* 12:139-42, 1963. Which-bone from first column of page 141.

J. Fourcade and M. Caron: Sur une série dramatique d'intoxications saturnines d'origine hydrique: *Ann. de méd. légale et de crim.* 34: 191-6, 154.

D. A. Henderson and J. A. Inglis: Lead Content of Bone in Chronic Bright's Disease: *Australian Annals of Medicine.* 6:145-54, 1957. Which-bone from Tables 1 and II, omitting infants.

Z. Jaworowski: Stable Lead in Fossil Ice and Bones: *Nature.* 217:152, 3.

R. A. Kehoe: *Metabolism of Lead in Man in Health and Disease*, 1961, 81 pp., Table 16, or in Harben Lectures, 1960; Table 16. Also in *Journal of Royal Institute of Public Health and Hygiene*, 1961, p. 93.

A. Maulbetsch and E. Rutishauser: La Teneur des dents en plomb; *Archives International de Pharmacodynamie et de Therap.* 53:55-64, 1936.

A. S. Minot and J. C. Aub: Distribution of Lead in the Human Organism: *Journal of Industrial Hygiene.* 6:149-58; cases from pp. 154-6.

R. E. Nusbaum, E. M. Butt, T. C. Gilmour, and S. L. DiDio: Relation of Air Pollutants to Trace Metals in Bone: *Arch. Environmental Health.* 10:227-32, 1965, Table 6.

Henry A. Schroeder and Isabel H. Tipton: The Human Body Burden of Lead: *Arch. of Environmental Health.* 17:965-78, 1968, Table 3.

C. D. Stehlow and T. J. Kneip: Distribution of Lead and Zinc in the Human Skeleton: *American Industrial Hygiene Association Journal.* 30:372-8, 1969, Tables I and II.

S. L. Tompsett: Determination and Distribution of Lead and Zinc in the Human Tissues and Excreta: *Analyst.* 8:330-9, 1956; Table IV.

S. L. Tompsett: Distribution of Lead in Human Bones: *Biochem. Jol.* 30:345 ff., 1936; Table 1.

S. L. Tompsett and A. B. Anderson: Lead Content of Human Tissues and Excreta: *Biochem. Journal.* 29:1851-64, 1935; Table II.

E. Weinig and B. Börner: Ueber den normalen Bleigehalt der menschlichen Knochen: *Archiv Toxicol.* 19:34 ff., 1961; Table 4.

F. Weyrauch and H. Müller: Ueber den Bleigehalt in Organen und Knochen bei bleikranken und bleigefärdeten Menschen: *Archiv fur Hyg. und Bakter.* 114:46-55; Table 3.

Appendix D

New Interpretations of History

Our study of ancient lead poisoning should serve not only to shed a truer light on Roman history, but to show possibilities of reinterpreting all history thru the use of medical, chemical, biological, and other sciences. To illustrate this, let us take the parallel case of Darwinism. We all know what a profound effect the theory of evolution has had on views of biologic and world history. Did it require a colossal genius like Darwin to do all that? Not exactly: you or I, or many of us together, might have perceived it. History shows that Darwin had several predecessors and a contemporary rival in Wallace. Any educated gentleman of 1859 could have created and proved the whole Darwinian doctrine if he had only reasoned naturally from the following five propositions already familiar to him:

1. Offspring tend to resemble their parents.
2. But offspring differ somewhat.
3. Some inborn qualities promote and some hinder survival, thru death, mating and/or fecundity.
4. Races have been deliberately and profoundly modified by breeders.
5. The animals and plants have been classified by biologists into varieties (species, genera, classes, etc.) according to their degrees of similarity.

That is all, logically, that Darwin needed to know. His voyage in the *Beagle* and all his patient experiments and studies could have been dispensed with, and were, by men who just thot straight, using the above five facts known in 1859 to all well-educated people.

Still, among all the people who perceived and mentioned these and their implications for evolution, none succeeded and brot about the intellectual revolution of evolution except Darwin. Why? Evidently because Darwin was the only man who had buttressed this great idea with a lifetime of observation, experimentation, and publication to ram this idea into people's minds, past all the obstacles posed by tradition, religious ideas, pride in being a man, not an animal. It was the *extra*, logically superfluous work that was really necessary—the overproof.

So as to new theories or laws of history, which we discussed in Chapter 14, Section 9, page 179, many have propounded them, some by much labor have gained some converts, but none has made them precise, proved, and preeminent like Darwinism.

Ellsworth Huntington, by genius and a lifetime of labor and study from the steppes of central Asia to the depths of statistics, established many a principle of human geography. Yet he found himself led ever more into questions of race, eugenics and dysgenics to explain what happened to the various nations. But he also accepted (see Geoffrey Martin's biography[1]) as a partial explanation for the differing histories of nations the Law of Coldward Progress, as demonstrated by an obscure young fellow he named, who was Gilfillan, and well rewarded him for it by a lifetime of friendship.

This law proposes that civilization began in very hot countries (Mesopotamia and Egypt) and as it progressed its centers of highest leadership moved northward into progressively cooler regions until the collapse of Roman civilization and brain power, when the center of leadership moved suddenly warmward, to Carthage, Alexandria, and Antioch (but also Constantinople), and thereafter to Baghdad. As civilization gradually recovered, its *ridge isotherm*, its belt of highest development, again moved steadily coldward, until today it lies along the isotherm of 10°C (50°F) for the annual mean, about the line of New York, London, Paris, Munich, and Vienna, as the climate worsens inland by increasing extremes of temperature.[2]

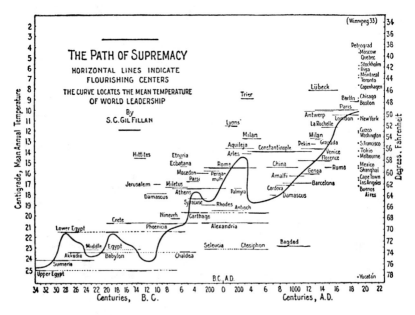

Huntington further showed the *frequency of cold fronts,* which bring thunderstorms and sudden drops of temperature and barometer, was also a requirement for highest vigor of civilization. The cold fronts which entail thunderstorms and sudden drops of barometric pressure, bring out air from underground that has been negatively ionized, a newly discovered factor, especially stimulating to children.

So only a few areas in the world, along that isotherm from our Great Plains to Vienna, met both requirements of thunderstorms and sudden drops in barometric pressure. Yet since Huntington's and my time, 1920, the advance of the Southern California coast, from San Francisco to San Diego, to rival the best in civilization altho having neither the $50°F$ mean nor cold fronts, has shown that a narrow range of temperature near the ideal can be a substitute. In Santa Monica on the ocean's coast in the Los Angeles conurbation, hardly a day in a year is too hot or too cold for comfort.

My first expression of this law was an article entitled The Coldward Course of Progress, in *Political Science Quarterly,* 35: 393-410, 1920, shortly afterward enlarged in *Historical Outlook,* 12:8-15, and echoed by Huntington's *Human Geography,* Kimball Young's *Source Book for Sociology,* Lynn White in C. F. Stover, ed., *Technological Order,* and by many another social geographic writer. The latest is L. D. Lambert[2] who gave us his copy of my cut, used by permission above. Herbert Spencer, I have found, had long ago expressed the idea of coldward progress in one perfect paragraph *(Principles of Sociology,* I: 18, 3rd ed.). But it takes more than one paragraph to establish a principle. And there have been other adumbrations, besides his and Huntington's.

1. Geoffrey J. Martin: *Ellsworth Huntington, his Life and Thought.* 373 pp., 1973, Archon Book, Hamden, CT 06514.
2. L. Don Lambert: The Role of Climate in the Economic Development of Nations, *Land Economics,* 47:339-344, 1971.

Appendix E   A Polyglot Glossary of Lead

ENGLISH	CHEMICAL	LATIN	GREEK	GERMAN	FRENCH
Barrel		Cupa, Vasa lignea	α	Fass, Tonne	baril
Bronze or copper	Cu; or Cu, Sn and Pb	AEs	Χαλκος	Bronze	bronze
Ceruse, cerussa, white lead	$2PbCO_3$, $Pb(OH)_2$ or lead carbonate and hydroxide	cerussa	Ψιμυθιον	Bleiweiss	céruse
Fermenting vat		dolium	πιθος		
Galena, lead sulfide, lead-glance	PbS	galena		Bleiglanz	galène
Grape syrup		Sapa, defrutum, carenum, caroenum	ξψηχα, καρουναχ σφειον	Moste	sabe
Lead	Pb	Plumbum, plumbum nigrum	μολυβδος, μολυβος	Blei	plomb

English	Formula	Latin	Greek	German	French
Lead glance, Lead oxide—see minium	PbS				
Litharge	PbO	Lithargurium	$\lambda\iota\theta\alpha\rho\gamma\upsilon\rho o\varsigma$	Bleiglätte	litharge
Minium	Pb_3O_4, Lead oxide	minium	$\sigma\alpha\nu\delta\upsilon\xi$	Mennige	minium
Must, unfermented grape juice		mustum	$\gamma\lambda\epsilon\upsilon\kappa o\varsigma$, $\tau\rho\upsilon\xi$	Most	moût
Pewter	Pb and Sn	no equivalent		Hartzinn	potée d'étain, étain
Red lead—see minium					
Sugar of lead	$Pb(C_2H_3O_2)_2$, lead acetate	Plumbum aceticum			
Tin	Sn	Stannum, stagnum plumbum album	$\kappa\alpha\sigma\sigma\iota\tau\epsilon\rho o\varsigma$	Zinn	étain

White lead—see Ceruse, and L. G. Stevenson: on the meaning of the words Cerussa and Psimithium: *Journal of the History of Medicine and Allied Science.* And Stevenson,* p. 33 N, 141, cites various ancient uses of terms.

Appendix F

Our Starred* References

Following is a list of books or articles of particular usefulness for our studies, and/or of frequent citation.

Apicius: *The Roman Cookery Book*, a critical translation of his *Art of Cooking:* by Barbara Flower and Elizabeth Rosenbaum, G. G. Harrap pub., London, 1958, 240 pp. Includes Latin original, translation, discussion, and seven pp. by Joan Liversidge on Roman Kitchens and Cooking Utensils. Three-fifths of the original was on luxury dishes of the first century A.D., and the rest on cheaper dishes was added in the 4th or 5th century A.D., 478 recipes, with no mentions but many indications of lead. Four halftones of ancient pots and utensils.

Athenaeus of Naucratis, Egypt, around 200 A.D.: *Deipnosophistae*, or *Savants of the Table*, with much on luxurious eating. Translation from the Greek.

Bernstein, Marianne: Techniques of Stratified Sampling in the Study of Variation of the Human Sex Ratio: *Eugenics Qly.*, 14:54-9, 1967. Supplies the sex ratios of the offspring of men of different professions, showing wide differences. Baldness also is especially characteristic of the son-begetting men.

Brothwell, Don R.: *Digging Up Bones*, the excavation, treatment and study of human skeletal remains. By a Curator in the British Museum, London, which pub. it in 1963, 210 pp.

Cantarow, Ab., and Max Trumper: *Lead Poisoning*, 1944, 6th ed., 1962 cited. Pub. by Saunders of Phila., 766 pp., a standard work.

Carcopino, Jerome: *Daily Life in Ancient Rome*, 342 pp., 1941, tr. from his *La Vie Quotidienne à Rome à l'Apogée de l'Empire*, 1939.

Cato, Marcus Porcius, the Elder, or the Censor, 234-149 B.C., his *De Re Rustica* or *De Agriculture*, in various translations.

Columella, L. J. M.: *De Re Rustica* (on Agriculture), about the mid-first century A.D. A native of Gades (Cádiz), who came to Italy. Much on viniculture, esp. in Book XII. Various translations, including that in *Les Agronomes Latins*, cited at the end of this Appendix.

Dioscorides, Pedanios, ca. 60 A.D., author of *(De) Materia Medica* or *Alexipharmica* or *Greek Herbal*; esp. about medicinal plants.

Forbes, Robert J., a prolific but not always accurate writer on ancient technics, who ignored lead poisoning except among lead workers and from pipes, in his voluminous *Studies in Ancient Technology.* We have usually cited his first ed., 9 vols., 1955-64; the 2nd ed. is of 1964 ff., from Leiden, Heineman pub.

Graham, Robert K.: *The Future of Man,* 1970, Christopher Pub. Hs., North Quincy, Mass., 200 pp. A good history of the human and sub-human races, esp. from the viewpoint of intelligence, how developed and lost.

Hofmann, Karl B.: Die Getränks der Griechen und Römer vom Hygienischen Standpunkte: *Archiv für Geschichte der Medicin,* Bd. 6, 1883, pp. 26-40 and 269-88. The first good exploration of ancient lead poisoning. He was Prof. of Medical Chemistry in Austria. One may consult also his Das Blei bei den Völkern des Altertums, in *Sammlung gemeinverständlicher wissenschaftlicher Vorträge,* 20:42-90, in German type, unlike the printing of the *Archiv.* This was also pub. as a book in Berlin, 1885.

Kobert, Rudolf (or Edw. Rud.): Chronische Bleivergiftung im klassischen Altertume: in *Beiträge aus der Geschichte der Chemie,* dem Gedächtnis von Georg W. A. Kahlbaum, Leipzig u. Wien, 1909, pp. 102-19. An excellent treatment of ancient lead poisoning, tho incited by Hofmann's and far exceeded by Stevenson's* unpub. thesis. But all missed the class angle.

Lead: Airborne Lead in Perspective; from the U. S. Natl. Acad. of Sciences, Com'ee. on Biologic Effects of Atmospheric Pollutants; 1972, 330 pp. incl. 600 citations.

Patterson, Clair C.: Contaminated and Natural Lead Environments of Man: *Archives of Environ. Health,* 11:344-60, 1965. Stresses that our present environment has about 100 times as much lead in it as the natural.

Patterson, Clair C.: Silver Stocks and Losses in Ancient and Medieval Times; *Econ. Hist. Rev.,* 2nd ser., 25:205-35, 1972. Supplies statistics of ancient lead production, by centuries.

Pliny, (C. Plinius Secundus, or Valerianus, or Pliny the Elder): *Natural History:* a vast encyclopedia of ancient knowledge and hearsay, dated about 77 A.D. Several times translated; the version by Bostock and Riley provides a general but poor index, while some other translations index only their particular volume. As usual when citing ancient writers, our citations refer to the Book and Chapter of the original, not to pages of the text, nor to any particular translation or original. Pliny lived near Vesuvius, and died in its eruption.

Soyer, Alexis: *The Pantropheon, or History of Food and its Preparation.* Lon., 1853, 474 pp. Rare, but in the Univ. of Calif. Agric. Lib. at Berkeley. Useful, tho it never seems to notice lead.

Stevenson, Lloyd G., MD, PhD: *A History of Lead Poisoning.* His doctoral dissertation in 1949, in 437 typed pages, with abundant footnotes. Photocopies of the whole or any parts may be obtained from the Eisenhower Library of Johns Hopkins Univ., Baltimore, MD 21218. An unparalleled history of lead poisoning, to which we have been greatly indebted, altho like all previous, it missed the class angle.

Tanquerel des Planches, L.: *Traité des maladies de plomb ou Saturnines:* Paris, 1839, 2 vols., 1,100 pp. Trans. into English in 1848, with a shortening to 441 pp. A very important work, which put together about all the essentials of lead poisoning known today, except chelating treatment, and added a rather competent history of the affliction and its understanding.

U. S. Environmental Protection Agency: *Biologic Aspects of Lead,* an annotated bib., 1972, 1500 pp. in 2 vols., covering 1950-64.

Waldron, H. A. & D. Stöfen: *Sub-clinical Lead Poisoning:* 224 pp., Academic Press, NY, 1974.

Wells, Calvin: *Bones, Bodies and Disease,* Evidence of Disease and Abnormality in Early Man; NY, Praeger, 1964, 288 pp.

Weyl, Nathaniel: Aristocide as a Force in History: *Jol. of Politics,* May 1967, and in *Intercollegiate Rev.,* June 1967, 9 pp.

Weyl, Nathaniel: *The Creative Elite in America,* 1966, 236 pp., Pub. Affairs Press, Wash.

Weyl, Nathaniel and Stefan T. Possony: *The Geography of Intellect.* Hen. Regnery pub., Chgo. 1963: 299 pp. An impressive demonstration of the unequal distribution of intellect in hundreds of parts of the world, and its explanations thru geography and history, with special attention to the leading regions.

Les Agronomes Latins, while this is not one of our Starred References, it is a handy set of volumes for anyone reading French, since it combines the agricultural (incl. vinicultural) writings of Cato, Pliny, Columella, Varro and Palladius, nearly all the Roman writers in thie field, in both Latin and French versions, Paris, 1864, under the direction of M. Nisard, 651 pp.

Appendix G
Data on the Author

He was born in St. Paul, Minnesota, 5.IV.89, the son of a missionary among the Ojibway Indians who originally came from Ulster; his mother was a minister's daughter of Connecticut Puritan stock. His autobiography, entitled "An Ugly Duckling's Swan Song," was requested and published in *Sociological Abstracts* in 1970 in forty pages. His undergraduate education, in languages and literature chiefly, was at the University of Pennsylvania, and his graduate training in Columbia University, New York, with an M.A. and Ph.D. in Sociology in 1920 and 1935. Altho he had tried architecture, his highest ambition, from 1910 to his last article in 1971 was to make long-range prediction scientific. This was reflected in his Master's essay at Columbia University, and in various articles, as outlined below.

From long-range prediction he moved into the social and psychological aspects of invention for most of the rest of his life, writing five books and forty articles on the subject. He also perfected from Ellsworth Huntington the Law of Coldward Progress of civilization's leadership (see Appendix D). He was a professor and a museum curator, and spent most of his life near the University of Chicago. He married an excellent wife, Louise, a social work executive who became his mainstay until her death 48 years later. But his investments paid off well, enabling him to put a lifetime into research and writing on the social aspects of invention.[1]

Before June 1938 he read a translation of Alb. Neuburger's *Technical Arts and Sciences of the Ancients* which had one of the few mentions in English of ancient lead poisoning (from Kobert*). Because of Gilfillan's rare life interest, the interface between the social and the physical sciences, and his concern for eugenics, roused by his most admired friend Huntington, he was able to perceive what all others had missed, the class angle of ancient lead poisoning. He sent a hundred-word summary of his argument to the American Sociological Society in May 1950, saying it would be the crown of his work. He later explained his idea also in Social Implications of Technical Advance, No. 4, vol. I of Unesco's *Current Sociology* in 1953. But presumably because of their attraction to the idea of human equality they cut this part out, except unmistakable references to it appear in the French summary.

213

In 1963, after finishing a book promised to the government on *Invention and the Patent System* that took him seven years, the author and his wife went to Europe to gather bones for clinical necromancy. But he was run over by an automobile in Messina, resulting in five fractures in his leg so had to return to the United States. They settled in Santa Monica, California, near his two children, Barbara (Mrs. John C. Crowley), now a lawyer of Pasadena with five children, and Marjorie Gilfillan who lives nearby. On his wife's death in 1971 the author re-visited Europe for more bones, and then settled near the University of California in Los Angeles for its library and luncheons at its Faculty Center, as well as to engage expert assistance on the present book.

The author just reached the age of 94 when he finished this book, and will be buried nowhere. His hopes of immortality are only that his discoveries will live on forever, his name in time forgotten, but truth is immortal. And his descendants will probably ever continue, unless all mankind be destroyed by dysgenic and/or atomic radiation.

(Editor's note: Dr. Gilfillan died on February 14, 1987, at the age of 97, while living with his daughter, Barbara.)

1. His Master's Essay, preserved at Columbia University, June 1920, was on the success of past long-range predictors whose prescience has been tested by time. His doctoral thesis was published in two books in 1935: *Inventing the Ship* and *The Sociology of Invention.* See opposite the title page for information on these two books, as well as all his other published books. His scientific articles that have been published are listed below, except for most of his earlier articles which are listed in his book, *The Sociology of Invention.*

The atomic bombshell, *Survey Graphic*, Sept. 1945, pp. 357-8. Anticipating the effects of atomic energy.

An attempt to measure the rise of American inventing and the decline of patenting. *Technol. & Culture*, I:201-214 and 227-234, 1960.

The coldward course of progress, in *Pol. Sci. Qly.*, 35:393-410, 1920, reprinted with amendments in *Hist. Outlook*, 12:8-15. Accepted by Ellsworth Huntington in his Temperature and the Fate of Nations in *Harper's Mag.*, 157:361-8 and in his *Economic and Social Geography*, Wily pub., 1933, pp. 141,2; and by Camille Vallaux, Franklin Thomas, Chas. Hodges, V. Stefansson in W. D. Wallis and Willey's *Readings in Sociology*, pp. 65-72 (Knopf pub., 1929). Also accepted by Lynn White in Stover, C. F., ed: The Technological Order, a symposium of 1962, originally published in *Tech. & Culture*, 3 No. 4, Fall 1962; and also reprinted in Davis & Barnes, *Readings in Sociology*, and widely reviewed.

Comment presenting our Graph 7 to 1955 on the First Seagoing Auxiliary (The Savannah) in *The Rate and Direction of Inventive Activity*, Proceedings of a conference in Minneapolis, 1960, Princeton University Press, 1962, pp. 83-85.

The furutre home theater (describing TV in 1912), in *Indep.*, 73:886-91 1912. Largely reproduced by W. Wallis, Next 125 years, *Am. Statistician*, 19:40-41, April 1965.

Invention as a factor in economic history, *Tasks of Econ. Hist.*, supplement to *Jol. Econ. Hist.*, 5:66-85, Dec. 1945. Reprinted in *Pat. Off. Soc. J.*, 29:262-288, and in J. T. Lambie & R. V. Clemence, *Econ. Change in America*, 1954, pp. 152-168.

Inventions and discoveries (during 1931 and '32); in *Am. Jol. of Sociology*, 37:868-75, 1932 and 38:835-44, 1933; reissued in volumes entitled *Social Change* (of 1931 and '32). Classified and discussed lists, of the most socially portentous inventions and discoveries, preceded by general discussions of the prediction of social effects, of which the second was reprinted in the *Pat. Off. Soc. J.*, 15:567-9.

The inventive lag in classical Mediterranean society, *Tech. & Culture*, 3: 85-87, 1962.

Inventiveness by Nation—A note on statistical treatment; in *Geog. Rev.*, 20:301-4, 1930. Reprinted in *Pat. Off. Soc. Jol*, 12:259-67. Discussed the comparative inventive rank of nations and adds the possibility that the patent lawyers in some small countries might encourage patenting abroad.

The lag between invention and application, with emphasis on prediction of technical change. Paper at Princeton Conference, 1951, 25 pp. The first and main part was published in *Rev. of Ec. & Stat.*, 34: 368-385, 1952.

Lead poisoning and the fall of Rome, *J. Occupational Medicine*, 7:53-60, 1965. This article and largely identical article, Roman culture and dysgenic lead poisoning, *Mankind Qtl.* (Edinburgh), 5:131-148, 1965, have been widely reviewed in scientific and popular journals of various countries.

Measuring Russian inventiveness, *Pat. Off. Soc. J.*, 33:328-333, 1951. Compares Russia's patents taken abroad with other nations' foreign patenting, for 1913 and for the Soviets' most assiduous year, showing a decline to one-fifth.

A new system for encouraging invention, *Pat. Off. Soc. J.*, 17:966-970, 1935.

On invention and eugenics, answer to Lincoln Day, *Columbia Univ. Forum*, Fall, 1960, p. 50.

Our archaic patent system, *New Republic*, 85:370, 1936.

The prediction of invention, *Tech. Trends & Natl. Policy*, 1937, W. F.

Ogburn, ed., pp. 15-23. On the techniques of prediction, as verified from past successful practitioners. Reprinted for Harvard use.

The prediction of technical change, *Rev. of Ec. & Stat.*, 34:368-385, 1962. Reprinted by Bright, J. R., ed., *Research, Development and Technologic Innovations*, Homewood, Ill., R. D. Irwin, 1964, with our 38 Principles.

The root of patents, or squaring patents by their roots. *Pat. Off. Soc. J.*, 31:611-623, 1949.

The size of future liners, *Indep. Mag.*, 74:541-543, 1913.

Social effects of inventions, in *Tech. Trends & Natl. Policy*, 1937, W. F. Ogburn, ed., reprinted in *Pat. Off. Soc. Jol.*, 1938, *Sci. Dig.*, Jan. 1938, *Think*, and reworked in Rosen, S. M. & Laura Rosen: *Technology & Soc.*, 1941.

A sociological study of inventors, *Pat. Off. Soc. J.*, 10:115-119, 1927. A critique of H. Hart. Preliminary conclusions from a study of inventors.

A sociologist looks at technical prediction, in *Technological Forecasting for Industry and Government*, J. R. Bright, ed., NJ, Prentice-Hall, 1968, pp. 3-34. A study of the methods of prediction, and of the most successful predictive writers, from their start, 1730-1950, with some attempt to measure their degrees of success, as proved by the event, and to correlate success with their methods, personality and subjects.

Some racial comparisons of inventiveness, *Mankind Qtl.*, 9:120-129, 1969, Much as in pp. 73-87, S. C. Gilfillan, *Supplement to Sociology of Invention*, 1971, San Francisco pub.

Some results of failure to foresee the effects of technologic change, *Soc. Sci.*, 21:172-181, 1946, accompanied by papers of others in that field.

An Ugly Duckling's Swan Song, the author's autobiography, *Sociological Abstracts*, 18:i-x1, 1970, and probably later in a book of sociologists' autobiographies.

Who invented it?, *Sci. Mo.*, 25:529-34, 1927. Reprinted in *Jol. of Pat. Off. Soc.*, 10:215-25 and W. D. Wallis and Willey's *Readings in Sociology*, pp. 65-72. (Knopf, 1929). Also published by Samuel Koenig *Sociology, a Book of Readings*, Hopper & Gross.

World projections for the air age, *Surveying & Mapping*, 6:12-18, 1946. Presenting my new "Matter-most map," as well as a doubly equidistant one centered on Paris and Chicago.

Dysgenic lead poisoning as the principal destroyer of ancient genius and culture, *J. Applied Nutrition*, 19:95-99, 1967; similar to my paper at the Third International Congress of Human Genetics, Chicago.

Appendix H

Repository of Our Materials

The Smithsonian Institution in Washington, the great national museum and center for anthropological studies, has agreed, thru the kindness of its distinguished curator, Dr. J. Lawrence Angel, appraiser of the personal ages of ancient Greek and Levantine bones, to store and make available for further studies Gilfillan's hundreds of ancient bones and fragments and his papers, books, and correspondence related to ancient plumbism, for use by further capable researchers. Only serious scientists should apply for such bones or documents.

The written and printed materials include the pertinent pages of Dr. Stevenson's* unequaled *History of Lead Poisoning*, in typescript, a brief study of our problem by George W. Nowell, a hundred or so of the books and pamphlet reprints we have most used, about 5,000 3x5 cards written or typed with abbreviations, the original reports from the laboratories, especially LCIT, and my complete correspondence on the study, a file of mostly typescripts extending lineally about half a meter.

217

Index